COSORI Air Cookbook 2022

By Dean Pearson

CONTENS

APPETIZER RECIPES 73

MEAT RECIPES.. 104

VEGETABLES RECIPES 121

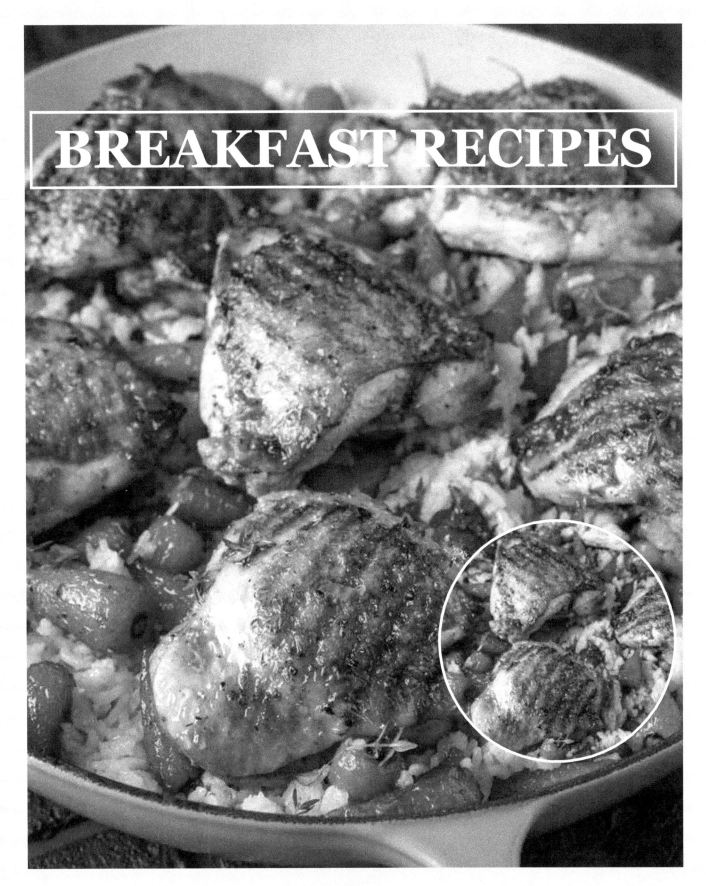

BREAKFAST RECIPES

Winter Sunshine Breakfast Galettes

Cooking Time: 4 minutes   Servings: 4

INGREDIENTS

√ 2 premade pie crusts
√ Flour, for dusting
√ 1½ tablespoons Dijon mustard
√ 1/3 cup creme fraiche
√ 1 cup white cheddar cheese, freshly shredded
√ 3 small white potatoes, cut into ⅛-inch-thick slices
√ 1 tablespoon olive oil
√ 1½ teaspoons kosher salt
√ 1 teaspoon black pepper
√ ½ teaspoon paprika
√ 4 large whole eggs, plus 1 large egg, beaten
√ 1 tablespoon fresh chives, chopped, for garnish
√ Flaky salt, for garnish
√ Items Needed:
√ Rolling pin
√ Pastry brush

DIRECTIONS

1. Roll the pie crusts out onto a lightly floured surface. Lightly smooth them out with the rolling pin, then cut 2 equally sized pieces out of each premade crust circle.

2. Roll the pieces out to make sure they are fairly round and quite thin.

3. Stir the mustard and creme fraiche together in small bowl, then spread an equal amount onto the center of each crust circle, leaving a 1½-inch border for the crust.

4. Sprinkle an equal amount of cheddar cheese on top of each crust.

5. Place the potatoes, olive oil, salt, pepper, and paprika in a medium bowl and toss to combine.

6. Arrange a layer of potatoes on each galette (about 12 to 15 slices), then fold the crust up over the edges to create a ruffle effect.

7. Brush the crusts of each galette with the beaten eggs.

8. Place the cooking pot into the base of the Cosori Indoor Grill, followed by the basket.

9. Select the Air Fry function, adjust temperature to 350°F and time to 12 minutes, then press Start/Pause to preheat.

10. Place the 4 galettes into the preheated basket, then close the lid.

11. Crack an egg on top of each when the timer ends.

12. Select the Broil function, adjust time to 4 minutes, and press the Preheat button to bypass preheating. Press Start/Pause to begin cooking.

13. Remove the galettes when done and transfer to a serving platter or plates.

14. Top each galette with fresh chives, then season with a pinch of flaky sea salt.

15. Serve immediately.

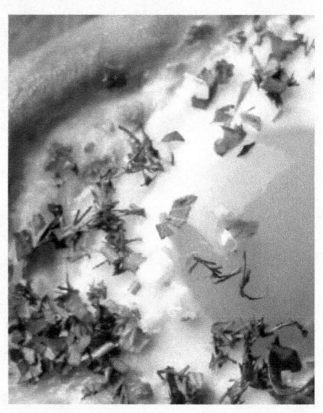

Pumpkin Spice Loaf

INGREDIENTS

√ ¾ cup pumpkin puree
√ 2 large eggs, room temperature
√ ½ cup light olive oil
√ ½ cup buttermilk
√ 1 teaspoon vanilla extract
√ ½ cup white sugar
√ ½ cup brown sugar, packed
√ 1¾ cups all-purpose flour
√ 1 teaspoon baking soda
√ ½ teaspoon salt
√ ½ teaspoon cinnamon
√ ½ teaspoon pumpkin pie spice
√ ¼ teaspoon ginger
√ ¼ teaspoon nutmeg
√ Oil spray
√ Maple Cream Cheese Glaze:
√ 1 package cream cheese (8-ounces), room temperature
√ ½ stick unsalted butter, room temperature
√ ¾ cup powdered sugar
√ ¼ cup pure maple syrup
√ 1 teaspoon vanilla extract
√ Pinch of salt
√ Chopped pecans or pumpkin seeds, for topping
√ Items Needed:
√ 2 mini loaf pans
√ Toothpicks
√ Stand mixer with paddle attachment

DIRECTIONS

1. Whisk together the pumpkin puree, eggs, oil, buttermilk, vanilla extract, and both sugars until smooth.
2. Add the flour, baking soda, salt, cinnamon, pumpkin pie spice, ginger, and nutmeg. Stir with a spatula until combined.
3. Select the Preheat function on the Cosori Air Fryer, adjust temperature to 300°F, and press Start/Pause.
4. Grease 2 mini loaf pans with oil spray. Pour the batter into the loaf pans, filling each 2/3 full. Make any leftover batter into muffins, if desired.
5. Insert the loaf pans into the air fryer baskets.
6. Set temperature to 300°F and time to 32 minutes, then press Start/Pause.
7. Remove loaves when a toothpick inserted into the center of each comes out clean.
8. Allow loaves to cool to room temperature before glazing.
9. Beat the cream cheese and butter in a stand mixer until smooth. Add the powdered sugar, maple syrup, vanilla extract, and a pinch of salt. Beat until smooth.
10. Glaze the mini pumpkin spice loaves with the maple cream cheese glaze and top with chopped pecans or pumpkin seeds.

Veggie Frittata

INGREDIENTS

√ 6 eggs
√ 3 green onions, chopped
√ ½ cup red bell pepper, chopped
√ 5 asparagus spears, chopped
√ 1 cup spinach, fresh
√ 1 tablespoon fresh basil, chopped
√ ¼ cup grated parmesan cheese
√ 1 teaspoon salt
√ 1 teaspoon black pepper
√ 3 tablespoons olive oil

DIRECTIONS

1. Heat a pan over medium-high heat. Add olive oil. Add chopped green onion, bell pepper, and asparagus. Season with salt and pepper. Sautee for 5 minutes.

2. Add spinach and stir until spinach wilts.
3. Remove from heat and allow to cool.
4. Whisk eggs and parmesan cheese in a separate bowl.
5. Add sauteed veggies and chopped basil.
6. Set the temperature on the Cosori Air Fryer to 320°F and press Start/Stop to preheat.
7. Pour mixture into a greased round 6x6 baking dish.
8. Place baking dish in preheated air fryer.
9. Cook at 320°F for 15 minutes.
10. Remove when Frittata is set and golden brown.

Matcha Mochi Pancakes

INGREDIENTS

√ 64 grams all-purpose flour
√ 64 grams mochiko flour
√ 1 tablespoon sugar
√ 1 tablespoon matcha powder
√ 2 teaspoons baking powder
√ ¼ teaspoon salt
√ 2 tablespoons unsalted butter, melted
√ 240 milliliters whole milk
√ 1 large egg
√ ½ teaspoon vanilla extract
√ Nonstick spray

DIRECTIONS

1. Whisk egg, milk, and vanilla together until light and bubbles form. Add flour, mochiko, sugar, baking powder, salt, matcha and whisk to combine. Fold in melted butter.

2. Add the pizza pan accessory pan (5-inch wide) inside the air fryer.
3. Select the Preheat function on the Cosori Air Fryer, adjust temperature to 180°C, and press Start/Pause.
4. Spray the pan with nonstick spray and add 32 grams of the batter to the pan.
5. Set time to 4 minutes and press Start/Pause.
6. Remove pancake and continue with the rest of the pancake batter.
7. Serve with your favorite toppings. Try layering them with fresh strawberries and butter on top!

Vegan Cinnamon Rolls

Cooking Time: 138 minutes   Servings: 8

INGREDIENTS

Dough
√ 1 cup unsweetened almond milk, slightly warm (100°-110°F)
√ ¼ cup vegan butter, melted
√ 2 tablespoon organic sugar
√ 1 teaspoon instant dry yeast
√ ½ teaspoon kosher salt
√ 2¾ cups all-purpose flour, divided

Filling
√ 6 tablespoons vegan butter, room temperature
√ 6 tablespoons organic dark brown sugar
√ 1 tablespoon ground cinnamon

Egg Wash
√ 2 tablespoons unsweetened almond milk
√ 1 teaspoon agave nectar

Glaze
√ 2 tablespoons unsweetened almond milk
√ ½ cup powdered sugar
√ ¼ teaspoon vanilla extract
√ Swedish pearl sugar, for sprinkling

DIRECTIONS

1. Whisk together the almond milk, melted butter, and sugar from the dough ingredients in a large mixing bowl.

2. Sprinkle the yeast into the milk mixture and allow it to bloom for 5 minutes.

3. Add kosher salt and 2¼-cups of flour into the milk and yeast mixture, then mix until well combined.

4. Cover the bowl with a towel or plastic wrap and set in a warm place to rise for 1 hour, or until it doubles in size.

5. Uncover and knead ½-cup all purpose flour into the risen dough. Continue kneading until it just loses its stickiness. You may need to add additional flour.

6. Roll the dough out into a large rectangle, about ½-inch thick. Fix the corners to make sure they are sharp and even.

7. Spread the softened vegan butter from the filling ingredients over the dough and sprinkle evenly with brown sugar and cinnamon.

8. Roll up the dough, forming a log, and pinch the seam closed. Place seam-side down. Trim off any unevenness on either end.

9. Cut the log in half, then divide each half into 8 evenly sized pieces, about 1½-inches thick each.

10. Line the food tray with parchment paper, then place the cinnamon rolls on the tray.

11. Cover with plastic wrap and place in a warm place to rise for 30 minutes.

12. Select the Preheat function on the Cosori Smart Air Fryer Toaster Oven, adjust temperature to 375°F, and press Start/Pause.

13. Whisk together egg wash ingredients and lightly brush the wash on the tops of the cinnamon rolls.

14. Insert the food tray with the cinnamon rolls at mid position in the preheated oven.

15. Select the Bake function, adjust time to 18 minutes, and press Start/Pause.

16. Remove when done.

17. Whisk together almond milk, powdered sugar, and vanilla extract from the glaze ingredients to make the icing, brush it all over the cinnamon rolls, then sprinkle the rolls with Swedish pearl sugar.

18. Cool before serving, or eat warm.

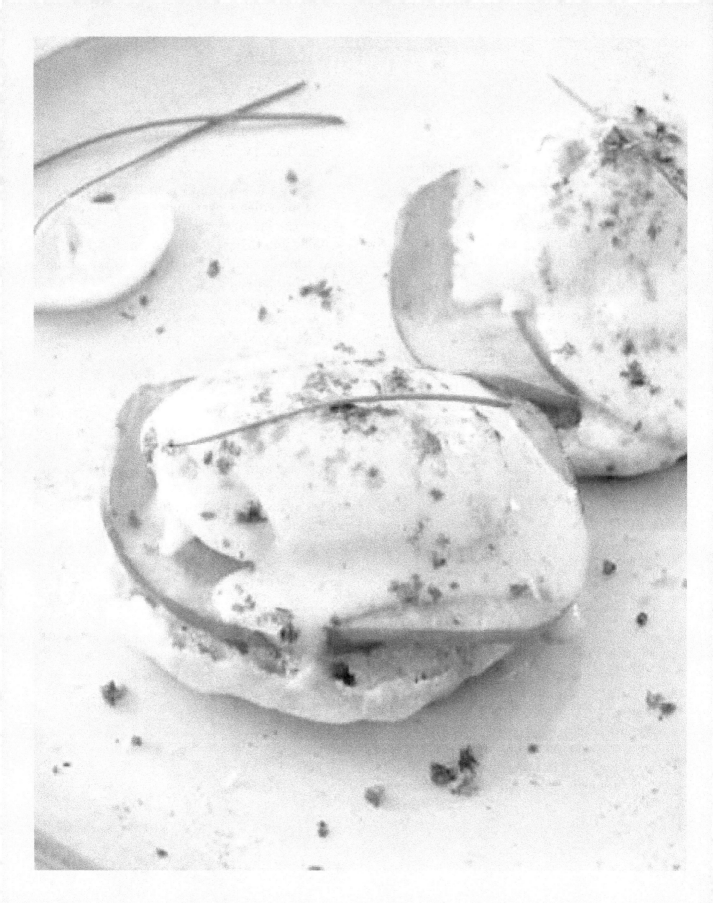

Eggs Benedict

INGREDIENTS

- √ 4 teaspoons grapeseed oil
- √ 16 tablespoons water, divided
- √ 4 large eggs
- √ 2 tablespoons of whipped salted butter
- √ 4 English muffins, sliced in half
- √ 8 slices Canadian bacon
- √ 1 large egg yolk
- √ ½ cup clarified butter
- √ TABASCO® Original Red Sauce, to taste
- √ 1 teaspoon Worcestershire sauce
- √ 1 lemon, juiced
- √ Kosher salt, to taste
- √ Chives, finely chopped, for garnish
- √ 1 teaspoon paprika, for garnish
- √ Items Needed:
- √ 4 ceramic ramekins
- √ Heat safe mixing bowl

DIRECTIONS

1. Brush each ramekin with 1 teaspoon of grapeseed oil.
2. Place 3½ tablespoons of water into each ramekin.
3. Crack one egg into each ramekin.
4. Select the Preheat function on the Cosori Air Fryer, adjust temperature to 310°F, then press Start/Pause.
5. Place the ramekins into the preheated air fryer.
6. Set temperature to 310°F and time to 10 minutes, then press Start/Pause.
7. Remove the ramekins when done.
Note: If the egg is not fully cooked, cook for an additional 2 minutes.
8. Drain the water out of each ramekin, being careful of the eggs.
9. Select the Preheat function, adjust temperature to 330°F, and press Start/Pause.
10. Spread whipped salted butter onto the English muffins, then place them into the preheated air fryer buttered side-up.
11. Set temperature to 330°F and time to 5 minutes, then press Start/Pause.
12. Remove the English muffins when done and set aside.
13. Place the Canadian bacon in the air fryer.
14. Set temperature to 330°F and time to 5 minutes, then press Start/Pause.
15. Remove the Canadian bacon when done and set aside.
16. Create a double boiler by filling a small saucepan 1/6 full of water, bringing it to a simmer, and placing a heat safe mixing bowl over the top.
17. Place the egg yolk and 2 tablespoons of water in the mixing bowl to begin the Hollandaise sauce.
18. Whisk vigorously until the egg yolk is fully combined with the water and the mixture is frothy.
19. Stream in the clarified butter slowly while whisking.
20. Continue to whisk until the sauce thickens, about 5 minutes.
21. Remove the mixing bowl from the double boiler and turn off the heat.
22. Whisk the egg and butter mixture vigorously until the sauce thickens further and begins to form soft peaks.
23. Add the Tabasco sauce, Worcestershire sauce, lemon juice, and salt, then whisk until well combined.
24. Taste the Hollandaise sauce and adjust seasonings to taste. Place the Hollandaise sauce in a warm area to prevent separation.
25. Assemble the Eggs Benedict by topping an English muffin half with 2 slices of Canadian bacon, a poached egg, and the Hollandaise sauce.
26. Garnish with chives and paprika.
27. Serve immediately with leftover English muffins on the side.

Strawberry Yogurt Parfait

Cooking Time: 1220 minutes   Servings: 6

INGREDIENTS
√ 4 cups whole milk
√ 3 tablespoons plain yogurt
√ Granola, for serving
√ Strawberries, sliced

DIRECTIONS
1. Place the milk in a pot and bring to a boil.
2. Cool the milk down to 115°F, then whisk in the yogurt until completely dissolved.
3. Cover the pot with a lid, set pot on the wire rack, then insert the rack at low position in the Cosori Smart Air Fryer Toaster Oven.
4. Select the Ferment function, adjust temperature to 110°F and time to 8-12 hours, then press Start/Pause. The longer you incubate the more tart the yogurt will be.
5. Remove the yogurt when done incubating and mix well.
6. Place the yogurt into the fridge with the lid on and refrigerate for 8 hours or overnight.
7. Assemble the parfait by placing granola at the bottom of a glass, followed by strawberries, then yogurt.
8. Top the parfait with more strawberries and granola.

Breakfast Blueberry Peach Crisp

Cooking Time: 70 minutes   Servings: 8

INGREDIENTS
Filling
√ 4 cups blueberries, fresh or frozen
√ 2 cups peaches, sliced
√ 1 teaspoon vanilla extract
√ 2 teaspoons lemon juice
√ 4 tablespoons pure maple syrup
√ 1½ tablespoons arrowroot
√ A tiny pinch of salt

Topping
√ 2½ cups rolled oats
√ 5 tablespoons almond meal (or almond flour)
√ 1 teaspoon cinnamon
√ 5 tablespoons pure maple syrup
√ 3 tablespoons coconut sugar (or brown sugar)
√ 7 tablespoons coconut oil, melted
√ 1 cup sliced almonds
√ 1 cup chopped walnuts
√ ¼ teaspoon salt

DIRECTIONS
1. Combine the blueberries, peaches, vanilla extract, lemon juice, maple syrup, arrowroot, and salt in a bowl and toss to combine. Pour mixture into the baking dish.
2. Combine all the topping ingredients in a separate bowl and stir until clumps form, then spread evenly over the fruit mixture.
3. Select the Preheat function on the Cosori Smart Air Fryer Toaster Oven, adjust temperature to 350°F, and press Start/Pause.
4. Place the baking dish on the wire rack, then insert rack at low position in the preheated oven.
5. Select the Bake function, adjust time to 1 hour, then press Start/Pause.
6. Remove crisp when golden on top and fruit is bubbly.
7. Serve with yogurt for breakfast or vanilla ice cream for dessert.

Spinach, Tomato, & Feta Quiche

Cooking Time: 278 minutes   Servings: 8

INGREDIENTS

Pie Crust

√ 1½ cups all-purpose flour, plus more for dusting

√ ½ teaspoon kosher salt

√ 3 tablespoons unsalted butter, chilled and cubed

√ 6 tablespoons vegetable shortening, chilled

√ 3 tablespoons ice water

√ Dry beans or uncooked rice, for filling

√ Filling

√ 1½ ounces frozen spinach, thawed and squeezed dry

√ 9 cherry tomatoes, halved

√ 1½ ounces crumbled feta cheese

√ 4 large eggs

√ ½ cup heavy cream

√ ½ teaspoon kosher salt

√ ¼ teaspoon freshly ground black pepper

√ Extra virgin olive oil, for drizzling

DIRECTIONS

1. Combine the flour and salt in a food processor and pulse once to combine.

2. Add the butter and shortening, then pulse until the mixture creates fine crumbs.

3. Pour the water in slowly and pulse until it forms a dough.

4. Form the dough into a square, wrap with plastic wrap, and place in the fridge for 6 hours or overnight.

5. Remove the dough from the fridge, unwrap it, and place onto a lightly floured work surface.

6. Roll out the dough into a 10-inch diameter circle. You may need to use additional flour to keep the dough from sticking to the rolling pin.

7. Place the dough into the tart pan and use your fingers to form the dough to fit the pan.

8. Trim the edges and prick the bottom of the tart shell all over.

9. Cover with plastic wrap and place in the freezer for 30 minutes.

10. Remove from the freezer, unwrap, and top with parchment paper that covers all the edges.

11. Fill the tart shell with dry beans or uncooked rice until the dough is fully covered. Set aside.

12. Select the Preheat function on the Cosori Smart Air Fryer Toaster Oven, adjust temperature to 350°F, and press Start/Pause.

13. Place the tart shell on the wire rack, then insert the rack at low position in the preheated oven.

14. Select the Bake function, press the Fan/Light button to start the fan, then press Start/Pause.

15. Remove the tart shell from the oven and let it cool for 1 hour.

16. Arrange the spinach, tomatoes, and feta cheese evenly inside the empty tart shell.

17. Whisk together the eggs, heavy cream, salt, and pepper until well combined.

18. Pour the egg mixture into the filled tart shell and lightly drizzle with extra-virgin olive oil. You may have some extra filling left over.

19. Select the Preheat function, adjust temperature to 350°F, and press Start/Pause.

20. Place the quiche on the wire rack, then insert the rack at low position in the preheated oven.

21. Select the Bake function, then press Start/Pause.

22. Remove the quiche from the oven and let it cool for 5 minutes.

23. Cut into slices and serve.

Asparagus Frittata

Cooking Time: 35 minutes   Servings: 4

INGREDIENTS

√ 3 tablespoons olive oil
√ 1 shallot, sliced
√ 18 asparagus spears, chopped
√ 1 teaspoon salt, divided
√ 1 teaspoon black pepper, divided
√ 6 eggs
√ 1 tablespoon fresh basil, chopped
√ 2 tablespoons grated parmesan cheese
√ 2 tablespoons shredded mozzarella cheese

DIRECTIONS

1. Heat a pan over medium-high heat. Add olive oil, shallot, asparagus, ½ teaspoon salt, and ½ teaspoon pepper. Saute for 5-10 minutes or until asparagus is tender. Place mixture into a bowl to cool for 5 minutes.

2. Whisk eggs, basil, parmesan, mozzarella, ½ teaspoon salt, and ½ teaspoon pepper. Add asparagus mixture and whisk until well combined.

3. Select the Preheat function on the Cosori Air Fryer, adjust temperature to 320°F, and press Start/Pause.

4. Grease the pizza pan with olive oil spray. Place mixture into the pan and insert into the preheated air fryer baskets.

5. Set, time to 20 minutes and press Start/Pause

6. Remove when frittata is set and golden on top.

Potato & Bacon Frittata

Cooking Time: 35 minutes   Servings: 4

INGREDIENTS

√ 2 slices bacon, chopped
√ 1 tablespoon olive oil
√ ½ onion, thinly sliced
√ 1 large gold potato, diced into ½-inch cubes
√ Salt & pepper, to taste
√ 6 large eggs
√ ½ cup grated Parmesan cheese

DIRECTIONS

1. Place the chopped bacon slices in a large nonstick skillet. Cook over medium high heat for 5 minutes or until the bacon is cooked and crispy. Move the bacon to a small plate.

2. Add olive oil to the skillet, then add the onion and potato. Season with salt and pepper. Sautee for 10-12 minutes, or until the potatoes are tender.

3. Remove from heat and place the bacon, potatoes, and onions into the greased baking dish.

4. Select the Preheat function on the Cosori Smart Air Fryer Toaster Oven, adjust temperature to 350°F, and press Start/Pause.

5. Whisk together the eggs, Parmesan, and a pinch of salt and pepper in a bowl. Pour egg mixture over the bacon, potatoes, and onions.

6. Place the baking dish on the wire rack, then insert the rack at mid position in the preheated oven.

7. Select the Bake function, adjust time to 15 minutes, then press Start/Pause.

8. Remove when the frittata is set. Allow to cool for 10 minutes before slicing.

Bacon and Cheddar Chive Scones

Cooking Time: 50 minutes   Servings: 4

INGREDIENTS

√ 8 slices bacon
√ 2 cups all-purpose flour
√ ½ teaspoon salt
√ 1 tablespoon baking powder
√ 2 teaspoons sugar
√ 4 tablespoons very cold unsalted butter, cut into small cubes
√ 1 cup shredded sharp cheddar cheese
√ 3 tablespoons freshly chopped chives
√ ¾ cup heavy whipping cream, plus more for brushing

DIRECTIONS

1. Select the Preheat function on the Cosori Air Fryer, adjust to 320°F, and press Start/Pause.
2. Place the bacon in the preheated air fryer basket.
3. Select the Bacon function, set time to 15 minutes, and press Start/Pause.
4. Remove the bacon when done cooking and cut into pieces. Set aside the pieces of cut bacon and reserve the bacon grease in two separate bowls.
5. Whisk together flour, salt, baking powder, sugar, and reserved bacon grease until well combined.
6. Cut the butter into the flour using a pastry blender or your hands until the mixture resembles coarse crumbs. Mix the cheddar cheese, bacon pieces, and chopped chives.
7. Fold the cream mixture into the flour mixture until it combines, then roll it out to 6-in x 6-in square.
8. Cut the dough diagonally two times making 4 scones and heavy cream on top of the scones.
9. Select the Preheat function on the Cosori Air Fryer, adjust to 350°F, and press Start/Pause.
10. Place the scones into the preheated air fryer basket lined with parchment paper.
11. Adjust the temperature to 350°F, set time to 20 minutes, and press Start/Pause. Flip the scones halfway through cooking.

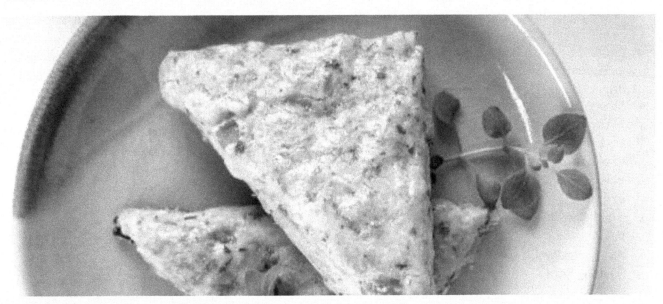

Asparagus Frittata

Cooking Time: 35 minutes   Servings: 4

INGREDIENTS

√ 3 tablespoons olive oil
√ 1 shallot, sliced
√ 18 asparagus spears, chopped
√ 1 teaspoon salt, divided
√ 1 teaspoon black pepper, divided
√ 6 eggs
√ 1 tablespoon fresh basil, chopped
√ 2 tablespoons grated parmesan cheese
√ 2 tablespoons shredded mozzarella cheese

DIRECTIONS

1. Heat a pan over medium-high heat. Add olive oil, shallot, asparagus, ½ teaspoon salt, and ½ teaspoon pepper. Saute for 5-10 minutes or until asparagus is tender. Place mixture into a bowl to cool for 5 minutes.

2. Whisk eggs, basil, parmesan, mozzarella, ½ teaspoon salt, and ½ teaspoon pepper. Add asparagus mixture and whisk until well combined.

3. Select the Preheat function on the Cosori Air Fryer, adjust temperature to 320°F, and press Start/Pause.

4. Grease the pizza pan with olive oil spray. Place mixture into the pan and insert into the preheated air fryer baskets.

5. Set, time to 20 minutes and press Start/Pause

6. Remove when frittata is set and golden on top.

Coffee Streusel Muffins

Cooking Time: 45 minutes   Servings: 6

INGREDIENTS

Crumb Topping
√ 1 tablespoon white sugar
√ 1½ tablespoons light brown sugar
√ ¼ teaspoon cinnamon
√ ¼ teaspoon salt
√ 1 tablespoon unsalted butter, melted
√ 3 tablespoons all-purpose flour

Muffins
√ ¾ cup all-purpose flour
√ ¼ cup light brown sugar
√ 1 tcaspoon baking powder
√ ½ teaspoon cinnamon
√ ⅛ teaspoon salt
√ ½ cup sour cream
√ 3 tablespoons unsalted butter, melted
√ 1 egg
√ 1 teaspoon vanilla
√ Cooking Spray

DIRECTIONS

1. MIX all the crumb topping ingredients together until it forms coarse crumbs. Set aside.

2. COMBINE together the flour, brown sugar, baking powder, baking soda, cinnamon, and salt in a large bowl.

3. WHISK the sour cream, butter, egg, and vanilla together in a separate bowl until well combined.

4. MIX the wet ingredients into the dry until well combined.

5. SELECT Preheat on the Cosori Air Fryer, adjust to 350°F, and press Start/Pause.

6. GREASE muffin cups with cooking spray and pour batter in until cups are ¾ full.

7. SPRINKLE the top of the muffins with the crumb topping.

8. PLACE the muffins into the preheated air fryer. You may need to work in batches.

9. COOK the muffins at 350°F for 12 minutes.

Soyrizo Breakfast Tacos

Cooking Time: 35 minutes   Servings: 3-4

INGREDIENTS
√ 1 large russet potato, skinned, cut into ½-inch cubes
√ ¼ yellow onion, chopped
√ ½ teaspoon garlic powder
√ ½ teaspoon black pepper
√ ¼ teaspoon salt
√ 2 tablespoons olive oil
√ 5 ounces soy chorizo
√ 2 eggs, beaten
√ Corn tortillas, for serving
√ Cilantro, for garnish
√ Queso fresco, for garnish

DIRECTIONS
1. Place the cake pan accessory in the Cosori Air Fryer basket.
2. Select the Preheat on the Cosori Air Fryer, adjust the temperature to 350°F, and press Start/Pause.
3. Mix the potato cubes, onion, garlic powder, black pepper, salt, and olive oil in a bowl.
4. Place the potatoes in the cake pan accessory in the preheated air fryer basket.
5. Adjust temperature to 350°F, set time to 20 minutes, and press Start/Pause.
6. Remove the air fryer basket and top the potatoes with the
7. Cook at 350°F for another 5 minutes.
8. Pour the eggs on top of cooked potato and chorizo and cook at 350°F for 5 additional minutes.
9. Serve on top of corn tortillas and garnish with cilantro and crumbled queso fresco.

Muffin Breakfast Sandwich

Cooking Time: 12 minutes   Servings: 1

INGREDIENTS
√ Cooking spray
√ 1 slice white cheddar cheese
√ 1 slice Canadian bacon
√ 1 English muffin, split
√ 1 tablespoon hot water
√ 1 large egg
√ Salt & pepper, to taste

DIRECTIONS
1. Spray the inside of a 3-ounce ramekin with cooking spray and place into the Cosori Air Fryer.
2. Select Preheat, adjust to 320°F, and press Start/Pause.
3. Add the cheese and Canadian bacon to 1 half of the English muffin.
4. Place both halves of the muffin into the preheated air fryer.
5. Pour the hot water and egg into the heated ramekin and season with salt and pepper.
6. Select Bread, adjust to 10 minutes, and press Start/Pause.
7. Take the English muffins out after 7 minutes, leaving the egg for the full time.
8. Assemble your sandwich by placing the cooked egg on top of the English muffin and serve.

Strawberry Rhubarb Scones

INGREDIENTS

√ 2 cups all-purpose flour
√ ¼ cup sugar
√ 2 teaspoons baking powder
√ ⅛ teaspoon salt
√ 1/3 cup unsalted butter, cold and cut into ½-inch cubes
√ ¼ cup rhubarb (fresh or frozen), finely chopped
√ ½ cup heavy cream, cold
√ 1 large egg, cold
√ 1 teaspoon orange zest
√ 1½ teaspoons vanilla extract
√ ¼ cup strawberries, finely chopped
√ 1 egg mixed with 1 teaspoon water, for glaze

DIRECTIONS

1. Stir together the flour, sugar, baking powder, and salt in a large bowl. Cut the butter into the flour mixture using a pastry blender or your hands until the mixture resembles coarse crumbs.
2. Whisk the heavy cream, egg, orange zest, and vanilla extract. Add the cream mixture into the flour mixture and stir until combined. Stir in the strawberries and rhubarb.
3. Select the Preheat function on the Cosori Air Fryer, adjust temperature to 360°F, and press Start/Pause.
4. Form the dough into ½-inch thickness on a lightly floured cutting board. Cut out the dough using a floured 2½-inch diameter biscuit cutter.
5. Line the preheated air fryer baskets with parchment paper.
6. Place scones onto the parchment paper, then lightly brush with the egg and water mixture and sprinkle with sugar, if desired.
7. Set the time to 13 minutes and press Start/Pause.
8. Remove when scones are lightly browned on top. Place scones on a wire rack to cool for 5 minutes. Serve warm by themselves or with your favorite jam or butter!

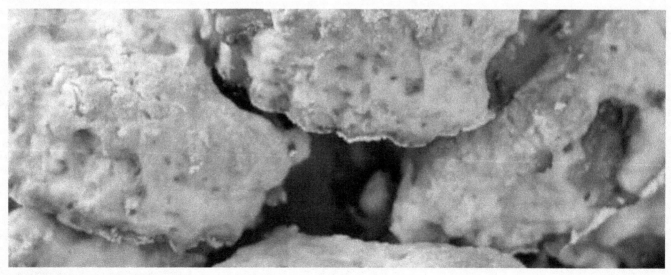

French Toast Sticks

INGREDIENTS
√ 4 slices white bread, 1½ inches thick, preferably stale
√ 2 eggs
√ ¼ cup milk
√ 1 tablespoon maple syrup
√ ½ teaspoon vanilla extract
√ Powdered sugar, for dusting
√ Cooking spray
√ 3 tablespoons sugar
√ 1 teaspoon ground cinnamon
√ 1/4 teaspoon salt
√ Maple syrup, for serving

DIRECTIONS
1. Select Preheat On The Cosori Air Fryer, Adjust To 350°F, And Press Start/Pause.
2. Cut A Slit In The Middle Of The Brioche Slice.
3. Stuff The Inside Of The Slit With Cream Cheese. Set Aside.
4. Whisk Together The Eggs, Milk, Heavy Cream, Sugar, Cinnamon, And Vanilla Extract.
5. Soak The Stuffed French Toast In Egg Mixture For 10 Seconds On Each Side.
6. Spray Each Side Of The French Toast With Cooking Spray.
7. Place The French Toast In The Preheated Air Fryer And Cook For 10 Minutes At 350°F.
8. Remove The French Toast Carefully With A Spatula When Done Cooking.
9. Serve Topped With Chopped Pistachios And Maple Syrup.

Baked Potted Egg

INGREDIENTS
√ Cooking Spray
√ 3 eggs
√ 6 slices smoked streaky bacon, diced
√ 2 cups baby spinach, washed
√ 1/3 cup heavy cream
√ 3 tablespoons Parmesan cheese, grated
√ Salt & pepper, to taste

DIRECTIONS
1. Select Preheat on the Cosori Air Fryer, adjust to 350°F, and press Start/Pause.
2. Spray three 3-inch ramekins with Cooking Spray.
3. Add 1 egg to each greased ramekin.
4. Cook the bacon in a pan until crispy, about 5 minutes.
5. Add the spinach and cook until wilted, about 2 minutes.
6. Mix in the heavy cream and Parmesan cheese. Cook for 2 to 3 minutes.
7. Pour the cream mixture on top of the eggs.
8. Place the ramekins into the preheated air fryer and cook for 4 minutes at 350°F, until the egg white is fully set.
9. Season to taste with salt and pepper.

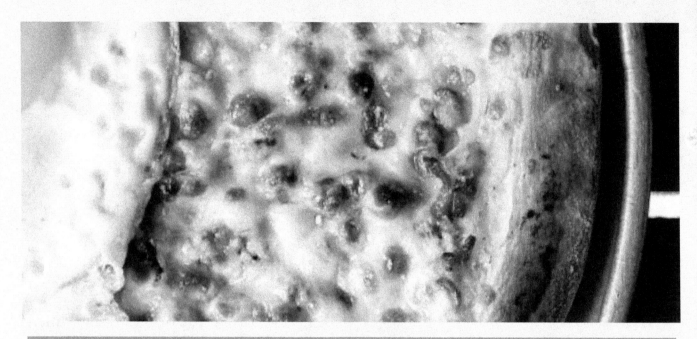

Berry and Apricot Flatbread

Cooking Time: 25 minutes   Servings: 4

INGREDIENTS
√ 1/3 cup whole milk ricotta cheese
√ 4 ounces mascarpone cheese
√ 4 ounces mascarpone cheese
√ ½ cup ricotta cheese
√ 2 tablespoons granulated sugar, divided
√ 1 egg
√ 2 tablespoons whole milk
√ 1 pre-packaged pizza dough
√ 3 tablespoons honey
√ 1 tablespoon hot water
√ ½ teaspoon vanilla extract
√ A pinch salt
√ Apricots, pitted and halved
√ Strawberries, sliced
√ Blueberries
√ Fresh thyme leaves, for garnish

DIRECTIONS
1. Mix together mascarpone, ricotta, 1½ tablespoons sugar, and vanilla extract until well combined. Store in the refrigerator.
2. Select the Preheat function on the Cosori Air Fryer, adjust to 350°F, and press Start/Pause.

3. Whisk together the egg and milk together to make an egg wash. Set aside
4. Cut the pizza dough to a 7 X 7 inch square.
5. Place the pizza dough into the preheat air fryer basket lined with parchment paper.
6. Brush the top with egg wash and sprinkle with ½ tablespoon sugar.
7. Adjust the temperature to 350°F, set time for 10 minutes, and press Start/Pause.
8. Combine the honey and hot water until the mixture is smooth. Set aside.
9. Remove the pizza dough when done cooking and allow to cool for 5 minutes.
10. Spread the sweetened cheese mixture onto the pizza dough.
11. Top with apricots, strawberries, and blueberries. Brush the top of the fruit with honey mixture and garnish with fresh thyme leaves.

Yogurt Bagels

Cooking Time: 40 minutes   Servings: 4

INGREDIENTS

√ 1 cup greek yogurt
√ 1 cup all-purpose flour
√ ½ tablespoon baking powder
√ ½ teaspoon salt
√ 1 egg, beaten
√ Toppings of your choice: everything bagel, sesame seeds, poppy seeds, zaatar, dukkah seasoning (optional)

DIRECTIONS

1. Combine the flour, baking powder, and salt in a bowl and whisk together. Add the yogurt and mix until combined and forms small crumbles.

2. Dust a work surface area with flour, remove the dough from the bowl, and knead the dough until it becomes tacky, about 20 turns.

3. Divide the dough into 4 equal sized balls. Roll each ball into ¾ inch thick ropes and join the ends to form bagels.

4. Brush each bagel with the beaten egg and sprinkle with seasoning of your choice.

5. Select the Preheat function on the Cosori Air Fryer, adjust temperature to 300°F, and press Start/Pause.

6. Line the fryer basket with parchment paper and place bagels into the preheated air fryer.

7. Set time to 20 minutes and press Start/Pause.

8. Flip bagels over and cook for 5 more minutes.

9. Let bagels cool for 15 minutes before cutting.

Ginger Blueberry Scones

Cooking Time: 26 minutes   Servings: 6

INGREDIENTS

√ 2 cups all-purpose flour
√ ¼ cup granulated sugar
√ 2 teaspoons baking powder
√ ⅛ teaspoon salt
√ 6 tablespoons butter, cold, cut into pieces
√ 1 teaspoon water
√ ½ cup fresh blueberries
√ 2 teaspoons fresh ginger, finely grated
√ ½ cup heavy cream
√ 2 large eggs
√ 2 teaspoons vanilla extract

DIRECTIONS

1. Sift together the flour, sugar, baking powder, and salt in a large bowl.

2. Cut the butter into the flour using a pastry blender or by hand until the mixture resembles coarse crumbs.

3. Mix the blueberries and ginger into the flour mixture. Set aside.

4. Whisk together the heavy cream, 1 egg, and the vanilla extract in a separate bowl.

5. Fold the cream mixture into the flour until it combines.

6. Form the dough into a round shape with 1½-inch thickness and cut it into eighths.

7. Brush the scones with an egg wash made from 1 egg and the water. Set aside.

8. Select Preheat on the Cosori Air Fryer, adjust to 350°F, and press Start/Pause.

9. Line the preheated inner basket with parchment paper and place the scones on top.

10. Cook for 17 minutes at 350°F, until golden brown.

Blueberry Banana Oat Muffins

Cooking Time: 30 minutes   Servings: 9-12

INGREDIENTS

√ 2 cups rolled oats
√ 1 cup almond flour
√ ½ teaspoon salt
√ ¾ teaspoon baking soda
√ 2 large eggs
√ 1 teaspoon apple cider vinegar (can substitute with lemon juice)
√ 1/3 cup maple syrup
√ 1 teaspoon vanilla extract
√ 1 ripe banana, mashed
√ ½ cup any non-dairy milk (can substitute with regular milk)
√ 1 tablespoon coconut oil, melted (can substitute with butter or olive oil)
√ 1 cup fresh or frozen blueberries

DIRECTIONS

1. Line muffin cups with liners and spray the inside of the liners lightly with nonstick cooking spray.

2. Make oat flour by blending rolled oats in a high speed blender or food processor until very smooth and resembles the texture of flour. Measure out 1 ¼ cups of the oat flour to use.

3. Whisk together the eggs, maple syrup, vanilla, mashed banana, non-dairy milk, coconut oil, and apple cider vinegar until smooth. Add the oat flour, almond flour, salt, and baking soda. Add the blueberries and fold to combine.

4. Select the Preheat function on the Cosori Air Fryer, adjust temperature to 300F, and press Start/Pause.

5. Fill each muffin cup with the batter ¾ full.

6. Place the muffin cups into the preheated air fryer basket.

7. Set the time to 18 minutes and press Start/Pause.

8. Remove muffins when a toothpick inserted into the center comes out clean.

9. Transfer the pan to a wire rack to cool for 10 minutes. Remove muffins from the pan and allow to cool for 10 more minutes before serving.

Strawberry Cream Scones

INGREDIENTS
√ 2 cups all-purpose flour
√ ¼ cup granulated sugar
√ 2 teaspoons baking powder
√ ⅛ teaspoon salt
√ 6 tablespoons butter, cold, cut into pieces
√ ½ cup fresh strawberries, chopped
√ ½ cup heavy cream
√ 2 large eggs
√ 2 teaspoons vanilla extract
√ 1 teaspoon water

DIRECTIONS
1. Sift together the flour, sugar, baking powder, and salt in a large bowl.
2. Cut the butter into the flour using a pastry blender or your hands until the mixture resembles coarse crumbs.
3. Mix the strawberries into the flour mixture. Set aside.
4. Whisk together the heavy cream, 1 egg, and the vanilla extract in a separate bowl.
5. Fold the cream mixture into the flour mixture until it combines, then roll it out to a 1½-inch thickness.
6. Use a round cookie cutter to cut the scones.
7. Brush the scones with an egg wash made from 1 egg and the water. Set aside.
8. Select Preheat on the Cosori Air Fryer, adjust to 350°F, and press Start/Pause.
9. Line the preheated inner basket with parchment paper.
10. Place the scones on top of the parchment paper and cook for 12 minutes at 350°F, until golden brown.

Breakfast Pizza

INGREDIENTS
√ 2 teaspoons olive oil
√ 1 pre-made pizza dough (7 inches)
√ 1 ounce low-moisture mozzarella cheese
√ 2 slices smoked ham
√ 1 egg
√ 1½ tablespoons cilantro, chopped

DIRECTIONS
1. Brush olive oil on top of the premade pizza dough
2. Add mozzarella cheese and smoked ham onto the dough.
3. Select Preheat on the Cosori Air Fryer, adjust to 350°F, and press Start/Pause.
4. Place the pizza into the preheated air fryer and cook for 8 minutes at 350°F.
5. Remove baskets after 5 minutes and crack the egg on top of the pizza.
6. Replace baskets into the air fryer and finish cooking. Garnish with chopped cilantro and serve.

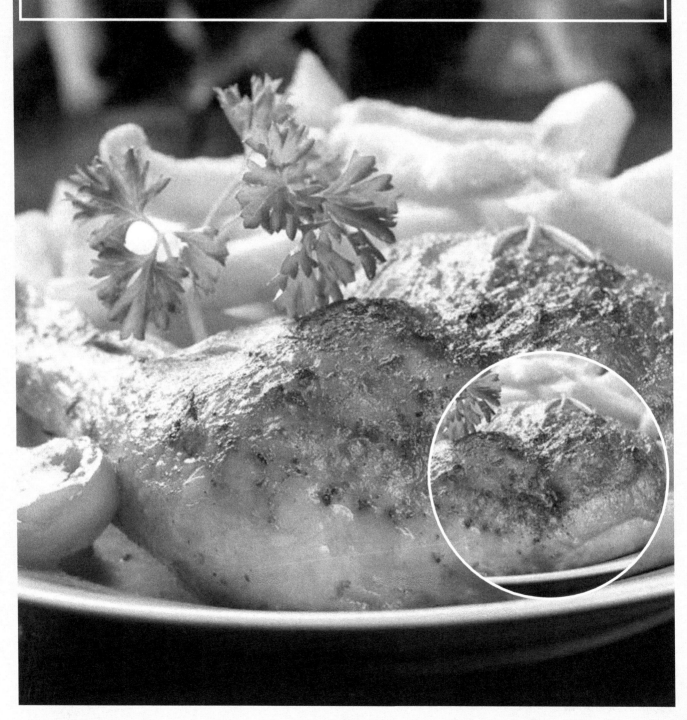

LUNCH RECIPES

Carnitas

INGREDIENTS

√ 3 pounds (1½ kilograms) pork butt or shoulder
√ 2 tablespoons (30 grams) orange zest
√ 7 garlic cloves, crushed
√ 1 large yellow onion, small diced
√ 1 serrano pepper, deveined and deseeded, cut into ¼-inch (6-millimeter) strips
√ 1½ teaspoons (8 grams) dried oregano leaves
√ 1 teaspoon (5 grams) ground cumin
√ 2 bay leaves
√ 2 teaspoons (10 grams) kosher salt, plus more to taste
√ 2 teaspoons (10 grams) ground black pepper
√ 1½ cup (354 milliliters) water
√ ½ cup (118 milliliters) fresh orange juice
√ 1 cinnamon stick
√ 12 small corn tortillas, warmed, for serving
√ Cilantro, chopped, for garnish
√ Onion, chopped, for garnish
√ Salsa roja, for serving
√ Salsa verde, for serving

DIRECTIONS

1. Trim any excess fat from the pork and slice into 4 equal portions. Discard any pieces of pure fat.
2. Combine the pork with the orange zest, garlic, onion, serrano pepper, oregano, cumin, bay leaves, salt, and black pepper.
3. Place the pork into the Cosori Smart Air Fryer basket, without the crisper plate.
4. Pour the water and orange juice over the top of the pork, add the cinnamon stick, then insert the basket into the air fryer.
5. Select the Roast function, adjust temperature to 375°F and time to 45 minutes, then press Start/Pause.
6. Flip the pork pieces halfway through cooking and stir the contents of the basket until evenly mixed.
7. Remove the pork when done and allow to rest for 10 minutes before shredding.
8. Serve immediately with tortillas, cilantro, onion, salsa roja, and salsa verde if desired as the main ingredient for a taco, burrito, rice bowl, or topping for a salad.

Simple Rack of Lamb

Cooking Time: 6 minutes   Servings: 2-3

INGREDIENTS

√ 4 ounces (113 grams) unsalted butter, softened
√ 3 tablespoons (45 grams) fresh rosemary, leaves only, minced
√ 2 tablespoons (30 grams) fresh parsley, minced
√ 4 tablespoons (60 grams) garlic, minced
√ ¾ pound (340 grams) rack of lamb, frenched
√ 2 teaspoons (10 millilitres) extra virgin olive oil
√ 4 teaspoons (20 grams) kosher salt, plus more as needed
√ 3 teaspoons (15 grams) ground black pepper, plus more as needed

Items Needed:
√ Electric hand mixer

DIRECTIONS

1. Whip the butter in a medium bowl using an electric hand mixer until soft and fluffy, about 3 minutes.

2. Fold the rosemary, parsley, and garlic into the butter, then set aside once fully combined.

3. Rub the rack of lamb with extra virgin olive oil, then season with salt and pepper.

4. Massage the herbed butter gently all over the rack of lamb, including in between the frenched bones.

5. Place the lamb directly into the Cosori Smart Air Fryer basket, without the crisper plate.

6. Select the Roast function, adjust temperature to 365°F and time to 6 minutes, then press Start/Pause.

7. Remove the lamb when done and allow to rest for 5 minutes.

8. Slice the rack of lamb and serve immediately.

Buffalo Chicken Wings

Cooking Time: 18 minutes   Servings: 3-4

INGREDIENTS

√ 1 cup Frank's RedHot® Original Cayenne Pepper Hot Sauce
√ ¼ cup of melted unsalted butter
√ 2 teaspoons kosher salt, divided
√ 2 teaspoons lemon juice
√ 1 pound chicken wings
√ 1 teaspoon grapeseed oil
√ 1 teaspoon ground black pepper
√ Oil spray
√ Ranch or blue cheese dressing, for serving
√ Carrot sticks, for serving

DIRECTIONS

1. Combine the hot sauce, melted butter, 1 teaspoon of salt, and lemon juice to make the buffalo sauce, then set aside.

2. Toss the chicken wings with grapeseed oil, remaining 1 teaspoon salt, and black pepper.

3. Select the Preheat function on the Cosori Air Fryer, adjust temperature to 380°F, then press Start/Pause.

4. Spray the preheated inner basket with oil spray, then place the chicken wings into the preheated air fryer.

5. Select the Chicken function, adjust time to 18 minutes, press Shake, then press Start/Pause.

6. Flip the chicken wings halfway through cooking. The Shake Reminder will let you know when.

7. Remove the wings when done and toss with the buffalo sauce.

8. Serve with ranch or blue cheese dressing, carrot sticks, and celery sticks.

Classic Margherita Pizza

INGREDIENTS

Homemade Pizza Dough:
- √ 1¾ cups bread flour, plus more for kneading
- √ ½ teaspoon granulated sugar
- √ 1⅛ teaspoons instant dry yeast
- √ 1 teaspoon kosher salt
- √ ¾ cup warm water (90°–110°F)
- √ 1 tablespoon plus 1 teaspoon olive oil

Items Needed:
- √ Stand mixer with dough hook attachment
- √ Food processor or blender

Tomato Sauce:
- √ 1 can peeled whole San Marzano tomatoes (28-ounces)
- √ 1½ tablespoons extra virgin olive oil
- √ ½ teaspoon kosher salt
- √ ¼ teaspoon dried oregano

Pizza:
- √ 1 premade pizza dough
- √ 1 tablespoon olive oil
- √ 6 tablespoons tomato sauce
- √ 1.5 ounces fresh mozzarella
- √ 8–10 fresh basil leaves, roughly torn

DIRECTIONS

Homemade Pizza:

1. Combine the flour, sugar, yeast, and salt in the bowl of a stand mixer with the dough hook attached and mix on low speed until well combined.

2. Add the warm water and 1 tablespoon olive oil and beat until the dough forms a ball, about 5 minutes.

3. Scrape the dough onto a lightly floured surface and gently knead into a smooth, firm ball.

4. Grease a large bowl with the remaining 1 teaspoon olive oil.

5. Add the dough, cover the bowl, and allow to rise until doubled in size. This will take about 1 hour, depending on the temperature of your kitchen.

6. Turn the dough out onto a lightly floured surface and divide into 2 equal pieces.

7. Cover each with a clean kitchen towel and let rest for 10 minutes before making your pizza.

Classic Margherita Pizza:

8. Drain the tomatoes and reserve the liquid.

9. Place the tomatoes, olive oil, salt, and oregano in a food processor or blender and blend until smooth. Season to

Note: Sauce will last 1 week in the refrigerator.

10. Select the Preheat function on the Cosori Air Fryer and press Start/Pause.

11. Stretch out the pizza dough into a 7-inch circle on a floured surface.

12. Place the pizza dough into the preheated air fryer. Brush the top with 1 tablespoon olive oil.

13. Set temperature to 400°F and time to 5 minutes, then press Start/Pause.

14. Flip the pizza dough over when the timer goes off and cook at 400°F for an additional 2 minutes.

15. Flip the pizza dough back over when the timer goes off and top with 2 to 3 tablespoons tomato sauce. Use the back of a spoon to spread it evenly across the surface, leaving ½-inch of space around the edge of the crust.

16. Break half of the mozzarella into large pieces and gently place them on top of the sauce.

17. Cook at 400°F for an additional 5 minutes.

18. Remove when the dough is golden brown and the cheese is melted.

19. Top with fresh basil and serve.

BBQ Chicken Pizza

INGREDIENTS

Homemade Pizza Dough:
√ 1¾ cups bread flour, plus more for kneading
√ ½ teaspoon granulated sugar
√ 1⅛ teaspoons instant dry yeast
√ 1 teaspoon kosher salt
√ ¾ cup warm water (90°–110°F)
√ 1 tablespoon plus 1 teaspoon olive oil
√ Items Needed:
√ Stand mixer with dough hook attachment

Pizza:
√ 1 large chicken breast, cooked and shredded
√ 1 cup spicy barbecue sauce, divided
√ 1 premade pizza dough
√ 1 tablespoon olive oil
√ 1 cup shredded mozzarella cheese
√ ½ cup shredded smoked gouda cheese
√ ¼ cup red onion, thinly sliced
√ 2 tablespoons fresh cilantro, chopped, for topping

DIRECTIONS

Homemade Pizza:
1. Combine the flour, sugar, yeast, and salt in the bowl of a stand mixer with the dough hook attached and mix on low speed until well combined.

2. Add the warm water and 1 tablespoon olive oil and beat until the dough forms a ball, about 5 minutes.

3. Scrape the dough onto a lightly floured surface and gently knead into a smooth, firm ball.

4. Grease a large bowl with the remaining 1 teaspoon olive oil.

5. Add the dough, cover the bowl, and allow to rise until doubled in size. This will take about 1 hour, depending on the temperature of your kitchen.

6. Turn the dough out onto a lightly floured surface and divide into 2 equal pieces.

7. Cover each with a clean kitchen towel and let rest for 10 minutes before making your pizza.

BBQ Chicken Pizza:
8. Select the Preheat function on the Cosori Air Fryer, then press Start/Pause.

9. Place the shredded chicken breast into a medium bowl. Add ½ cup barbecue sauce and toss to combine.

10. Stretch out the pizza dough into a 7-inch circle on a floured surface.

11. Place the pizza dough into the preheated air fryer. Brush the top with olive oil.

12. Set temperature to 400°F and time to 5 minutes, then press Start/Pause.

13. Flip the pizza dough over when the timer goes off and cook at 400°F for an additional 2 minutes.

14. Flip the pizza dough back over when the timer goes off and top with the remaining barbeque sauce, shredded chicken, shredded mozzarella and gouda, and red onion.

15. Cook at 400°F for an additional 5 minutes.

16. Remove when the dough is golden brown and the cheese is melted.

17. Top with chopped cilantro and serve.

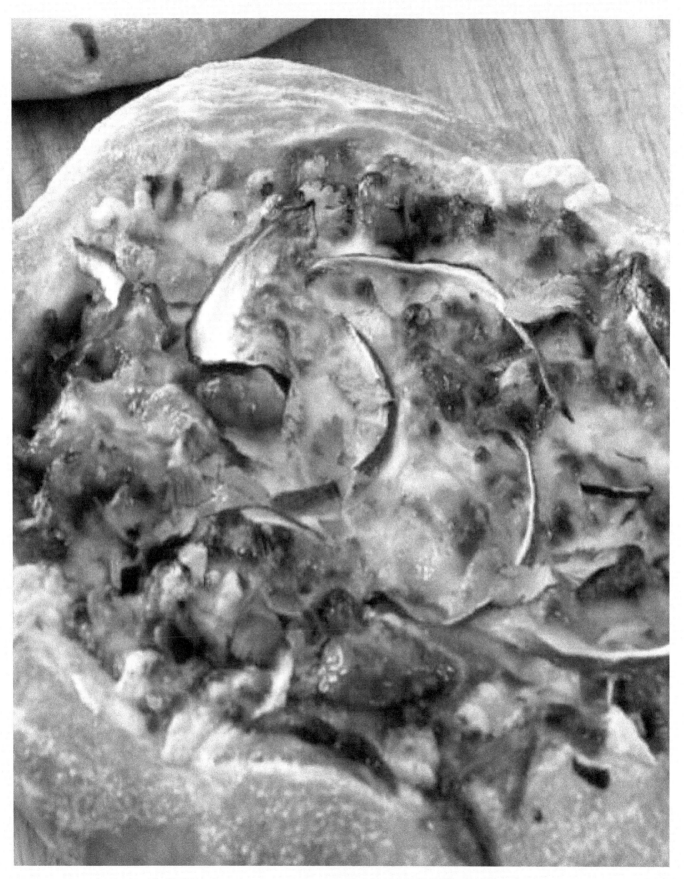

29

Guinness® Ribeye Steaks

INGREDIENTS

√ 16 ounces Guinness® (or any dark beer), flat and room-temperature

√ 5 garlic cloves, smashed

√ 3 tablespoons yellow onion, minced

√ 3 tablespoons soy sauce

√ 2 teaspoons Worcestershire sauce

√ 2 teaspoons dried tarragon

√ 1½ teaspoons Dijon mustard

√ 1 whole shallot, minced

√ 1 teaspoon dried parsley

√ 2 teaspoons ground black pepper, plus more for seasoning

√ 2 teaspoons kosher salt, plus more for seasoning

√ 2 ribeye steaks (8 ounces each)

√ Oil spray

Items Needed:

√ Resealable plastic bag

DIRECTIONS

1. Mix all ingredients except for the steaks and oil spray together in a large bowl to make the marinade.

2. Place the steaks and marinade into a large resealable plastic bag and mix well.

3. Marinate in the refrigerator for 8 hours or overnight.

4. Remove the steaks from the marinade, gently pat dry, then sprinkle both sides evenly with black pepper and kosher salt.

5. Place the cooking pot into the base of the Cosori Smart Indoor Grill, followed by the grill grate.

6. Select the Air Grill function on max heat, adjust temperature to 510°F and time to 7 minutes, press Shake, then press Start/Pause to preheat.

7. Spray the preheated grill grate with oil spray.

8. Place the steaks onto the preheated grill grate, then close the lid.

9. Flip the steaks halfway through cooking. The Shake Reminder will let you know when.

10. Remove from the steaks when done and set aside to rest for 5 minutes.

11. Serve the steaks immediately with your choice of sides.

Grilled Reuben Sandwiches

Cooking Time: 8 minutes   Servings: 2

INGREDIENTS

Dressing:

√ ¼ cup mayonnaise

√ 2½ tablespoons ketchup

√ ½ teaspoon Worcestershire sauce

√ ½ tablespoon grated horseradish, fresh

√ ¼ teaspoon Dijon mustard

√ 1 teaspoon white sugar

√ Kosher salt, to taste

√ Ground black pepper, to taste

√ 2 teaspoons cornichons, minced (optional)

√ 2 teaspoons yellow onion, minced (optional)

Sandwiches:

√ 4 slices rustic rye or pumpernickel bread (1-inch thick each)

√ 4 tablespoons dressing, divided

√ ½ cup sauerkraut, drained, divided

√ ½ pound corned beef, thinly sliced, divided

√ 6 slices Swiss or Gruyère cheese, divided

√ Oil spray

DIRECTIONS

1. Mix all dressing ingredients together in a small bowl.

2. Spread ½ tablespoon of dressing on both sides of each slice of bread.

3. Squeeze out the excess moisture from the sauerkraut. Pat dry with paper towels and set aside.

4. Top 2 slices of bread with ¼ pound of corned beef, ¼ cup of sauerkraut, and 3 slices of cheese. Finish by placing the last 2 slices of rye bread on top.

5. Place the cooking pot into the base of the Cosori Smart Indoor Grill, followed by the grill grate.

6. Select the Air Grill function on medium heat, adjust temperature to 425°F and time to 8 minutes, press Shake, then press Start/Pause to preheat.

7. Spray the preheated grill grate with oil spray.

8. Place the sandwiches onto the preheated grill grate, gently press down on each closed faced sandwich using a spatula, then close the lid.

9. Flip the sandwiches halfway through cooking, and press down again on each sandwich using a spatula. The Shake Reminder will let you know when.

10. Remove the sandwiches when done, let cool for 2 minutes, then slice in half.

11. Serve the sandwiches immediately.

Sunny Side Burgers

INGREDIENTS

√ Oil spray
√ 2 teaspoons kosher salt
√ 1 teaspoon ground black pepper
√ ½ teaspoon onion powder
√ ½ teaspoon garlic powder
√ 1 pound ground angus beef
√ 4 sunny side up fried eggs, with runny yolks
√ 4 slices Munster cheese, or cheese of choice
√ 2 cups caramelized onion
√ 2 tablespoons mayonnaise
√ 4 Brioche burger buns, sliced
√ Boston bib lettuce, as needed
√ Tomato slices, as needed
√ 2 teaspoons crushed red pepper flakes, for garnish
√ Ketchup, for serving
√ Yellow mustard, for serving

DIRECTIONS

1. Combine the kosher salt, ground black pepper, onion powder, and garlic powder together in a large bowl. Mix the spices into the ground angus beef and then form into four quarter pound patties, about a ½-inch thick.
2. Place the cooking pot into the base of the Cosori Indoor Grill, followed by the grill plate.
3. Select the Air Grill function on max heat, adjust the temperature to 510F and cooking time to 7 minutes, press Shake, then press Start/Pause.
Note: This will yield a medium-rare burger.
4. Spray the grill grate lightly with oil spray once the grill is done preheating.
5. Place the burger patties onto the preheated grill grate and press Start/Pause. Flip the patties when the Shake reminder beeps.

6. Add the cheese to the patties when 2 minutes remain on the timer.
7. Remove when done and set onto a wire rack to rest.
8. Spread the mayonnaise over the insides of the sliced Brioche buns.
9. Select the Broil function, adjust time to 3 minutes, press the Preheat button to cancel the automatic preheat, then place the buns mayonnaise side down onto the grill plate. Press Start/Pause then close the lid to begin cooking.
10. Remove the buns when toasted and set aside until cool to the touch.
11. Assemble the burgers by topping the bottom halves of the brioche buns with lettuce and tomato, then place the burger patty on top followed by caramelized onions, then the sunny side up fried egg, sprinkle with crushed red pepper flakes, and finish with the top half of the bun.
12. Serve immediately with the condiments on the side and pair with hashbrowns or home fries, and fresh fruit.

Ultimate 7-Layer Dip

Cooking Time: 5 minutes   Servings: 10

INGREDIENTS

√ 5 Roma tomatoes, small diced
√ 1 red onion, small diced
√ 1 cup cilantro, chopped
√ 1 jalapeno, minced
√ 4 limes, divided and juiced
√ Kosher salt, to taste
√ Ground black pepper, to taste
√ 4 avocados, pits removed
√ 5 flour tortillas (burrito size, 10-inch)
√ Oil spray
√ 8 ounces shredded cheddar cheese, plus more for garnish
√ 1 can refried pinto beans (16 ounces), warmed
√ 1 can refried black beans (16 ounces), warmed
√ 2 cups shredded rotisserie chicken, warmed
√ 2 cups salsa con queso, warmed
√ 2 cups sour cream
√ 1 bunch scallions, finely chopped, for garnish
√ Chips, for serving

Items Needed:
√ Aluminum foil

DIRECTIONS

1. Toss the diced tomatoes, red onion, cilantro, jalapeno and juice of 2 limes together in a medium bowl to make the pico de gallo.
2. Season to taste with salt and black pepper. Reserve ¼ cup and set aside.
3. Mash the avocados in a medium bowl. Add the reserved ¼ cup of pico de gallo and the juice of the remaining 2 limes.
4. Season the guacamole to taste with salt and black pepper. Set aside.
5. Select the Preheat function on the Cosori Air Fryer and press Start/Pause.
6. Spray both sides of each tortilla with oil spray.
7. Cut a line through 4 tortillas, starting from the middle all the way to the right side.
8. Fold the cut tortillas into loosely shaped cones and place each one seam-side down into each corner of the preheated inner air fryer basket. The cones will unravel slightly, creating a bowl formation.
9. Sprinkle ¼ cup of cheddar cheese across the bottom of the tortilla bowl.
10. Place the 5th tortilla over the cheddar cheese.
11. Trim the tortillas sticking out of the corners of the air fryer basket, lining them up with the edges of the basket.
12. Lay an aluminum foil sheet down into the air fryer basket on top of the tortilla bowl, then place several balls of foil on top to help it retain its shape while cooking.
13. Place another sheet of foil on top of the foil balls and against the tortilla walls, creating a tent to prevent the air fryer balls from floating up while cooking.
14. Insert the basket into the preheated air fryer.
15. Set temperature to 400°F and time to 5 minutes, then press Start/Pause.
16. Remove the air fryer basket and place onto a heatproof surface when done cooking.
17. Detach the inner air fryer basket and carefully remove the foil tent and foil balls. Let cool completely.
18. Transfer the tortilla bowl to a serving plate.
19. Layer the refried pinto beans, refried black beans, pico de gallo, guacamole, shredded chicken, salsa con queso, and sour cream in order into the tortilla bowl.
20. Garnish with cheddar cheese and scallions.
21. Serve immediately with chips.

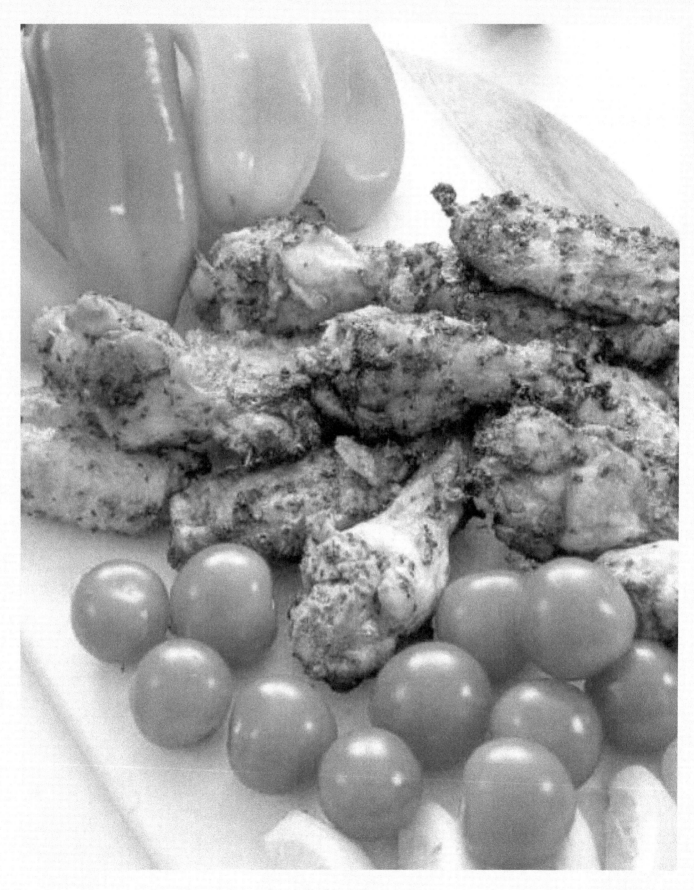

Lemon Pepper Chicken Wings

Cooking Time: 18 minutes   Servings: 3-4

INGREDIENTS
√ 1 pound chicken wings
√ ½ lemon, juiced
√ 2 teaspoons kosher salt
√ ¼ cup lemon pepper seasoning
√ Oil spray
√ Lemon wedges, for serving
√ Crudités, for serving

DIRECTIONS
1. Place the chicken wings, lemon juice, salt, and lemon pepper into a resealable plastic bag.
2. Marinate the chicken wings in the refrigerator for 15 minutes.
3. Select the Preheat function on the Cosori Air Fryer, adjust temperature to 380°F, then press Start/Pause.
4. Remove the chicken wings from the marinade.
5. Spray the preheated inner basket with oil spray, then place the chicken wings into the preheated air fryer.
6. Select the Chicken function, adjust time to 18 minutes, press Shake, then press Start/Pause.
7. Flip the chicken wings halfway through cooking. The Shake Reminder will let you know when.
8. Remove wings when done and serve with lemon wedges and crudités.

Teba Shio Chicken Wings

Cooking Time: 18 minutes   Servings: 3-4

INGREDIENTS
√ ¾ cup cooking sake
√ 1 pound chicken wings
√ 1 teaspoon kosher salt
√ 2 teaspoons Shichimi togarashi, plus more for serving
√ ¼ teaspoon freshly ground white pepper
√ 1 teaspoon grapeseed oil
√ ½ teaspoon lemon juice
√ Oil spray
√ Lemon wedges, for serving

DIRECTIONS
1. Place the sake and chicken wings into a resealable plastic bag.
2. Marinate the chicken wings in the refrigerator for 20 minutes, ensuring they are fully submerged.
3. Remove the chicken wings and pat dry with paper towels.
4. Season the wings with salt, Shichimi togarashi, white pepper, grapeseed oil, and lemon juice.
5. Select the Preheat function on the Cosori Air Fryer, adjust temperature to 380°F, then press Start/Pause.
6. Spray the preheated inner basket with oil spray, then place the chicken wings into the preheated air fryer.
7. Select the Chicken function, adjust time to 18 minutes, press Shake, then press Start/Pause.
8. Flip the chicken wings halfway through cooking. The Shake Reminder will let you know when.
9. Remove when done and serve with Shichimi togarashi and lemon wedges.

Hummus-Filled Portobellos with Olive Tapenade

INGREDIENTS

Hummus-Filled Portobellos:
√ 2 portobello mushrooms
√ 1 teaspoon olive oil
√ 1 teaspoon kosher salt
√ 1 cups prepared hummus
√ 1 teaspoon paprika

Items Needed:
√ Food processor fitted with blade attachment
√ Olive Tapenade:
√ 1 cup pitted kalamata olives
√ ¼ cup olive oil
√ 2 tablespoons capers, rinsed
√ 2 tablespoons fresh parsley, chopped, plus more for garnish
√ 2 garlic cloves, smashed
√ 1 lemon, zested and juiced
√ ½ tablespoon red wine vinegar
√ ½ tablespoon fresh oregano
√ ½ tablespoon fresh thyme
√ Kosher salt, to taste
√ Freshly ground black pepper, to taste

DIRECTIONS

1. Scrape out the gills underneath the mushrooms using a spoon and discard.
2. Brush the mushrooms caps with olive oil, then season with salt.
3. Fill each mushroom cap with hummus, then sprinkle paprika over the hummus.
4. Place the crisper plate into the Cosori Smart Air Fryer basket, then place the mushroom caps onto the crisper plate.
5. Select the Air Fry function, adjust temperature to 385°F and time to 12 minutes, then press Start/Pause.
6. Combine the olive tapenade ingredients in a food processor fitted with the blade attachment and blend until almost smooth, but some texture remains.
7. Season to taste with salt and pepper, then set aside.
8. Remove the mushroom caps when done.
9. Drizzle each mushroom cap with the olive tapenade, sprinkle with parsley, and serve.

Yuzu Ginger Chicken Skewers

INGREDIENTS

√ 1 pound boneless skinless chicken thighs, trimmed and cut into 1-inch pieces
√ 2 tablespoons bottled yuzu juice
√ ½ tablespoon yuzu kosho
√ 1 tablespoon tahini
√ ½ tablespoon lemongrass paste
√ 1 tablespoon grapeseed oil
√ 1 tablespoon sesame oil
√ 1½ teaspoons ginger, grated
√ 1 garlic clove, grated
√ 1½ teaspoons kosher salt
√ 2 green onions, thinly sliced, for garnish
√ Flaky sea salt, for garnish
√ Sesame seeds, for garnish

Items Needed:
√ 4 metal or wooden skewers

DIRECTIONS

1. Combine all the ingredients except the onions, flaky sea salt, and sesame seeds in a bowl and mix well. Cover and marinate at room temperature for 30 minutes.
2. Skewer the chicken evenly between the skewers.
3. Place the crisper plate into the Cosori Smart Air Fryer basket, then place the skewers onto the crisper plate.
4. Select the Steak function, adjust time to 10 minutes, then press Start/Pause.
5. Remove the skewers when done.
6. Garnish the skewers with green onions, flaky sea salt, and sesame seeds, then serve.

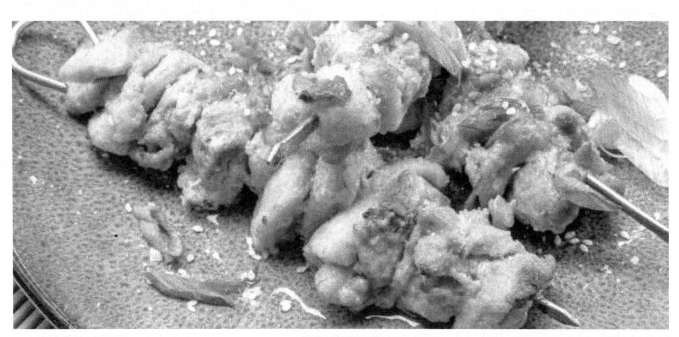

Korean BBQ

INGREDIENTS

Korean Short Ribs (Galbi):

√ ¼ cup soy sauce
√ ½ cup low sodium soy sauce
√ ¼ cup water
√ ⅛ cup rice vinegar
√ 1 bunch scallions, cut into 2-inch pieces
√ 5 mushrooms, quartered
√ 5 garlic cloves, smashed
√ ⅛ cup honey
√ 1 cup Assam pear puree
√ 12 ounces unsweetened apple sauce
√ 1½ pounds beef short ribs, cut Korean style
√ Oil spray

Pork Belly:

√ 1 pound thick-cut pork belly
√ 2 teaspoons kosher salt
√ 2 teaspoons ground black pepper
√ 1 head green leaf lettuce, washed, leaves separated for serving
√ Sesame oil, for serving (optional)
√ Coarse sea salt, for serving (optional)
√ Ssamjang (Korean soybean paste condiment), for serving (optional)
√ 1 bunch green onion, julienned lengthwise (cut into 2-inch strips, ⅛inch thick) for serving (optional)
√ White rice, for serving (optional)

DIRECTIONS

1. Place all the short rib ingredients except for the short ribs and oil spray into a large bowl and mix well.
2. Pour the marinade into a large resealable bag, then place the short ribs into the marinade.
3. Marinate overnight.
4. Remove the marinated short ribs from the marinade and gently pat dry with paper towels.
5. Season both sides of the pork belly pieces with the 2 teaspoons of kosher salt and 2 teaspoons of ground black pepper, then set aside.
6. Place the cooking pot into the base of the Cosori Indoor Grill, followed by the grill grate.
7. Select the Air Grill function on max heat, adjust temperature to 510°F and cooking time to 6 minutes, press Shake, then press Start/Pause.
8. Open the lid and spray the grill grate with oil spray once the grill is done preheating. You will need to work in 3 batches.
9. Place the short ribs onto the preheated grill grate, then close the lid to start cooking.
10. Flip the short ribs halfway through cooking. The Shake Reminder will let you know when.
11. Remove the short ribs when done and set aside.
12. Cut the short ribs with scissors, separating them evenly between each of the bones.
13. Repeat steps 9-12 for the remaining two batches of ribs.
14. Select the Air Grill function on max heat, adjust temperature to 510°F and cooking time to 8 minutes, press Shake, then press Start/Pause.
15. Open the lid and spray the grill grate with oil spray once the grill is done preheating. You will need to work in 2 batches.
16. Lay the pork belly pieces onto the preheated grill grate, then close the lid to start cooking.
17. Flip the pork belly pieces halfway through cooking. The Shake reminder will let you know when.
18. Remove the pork belly when done and set aside.
19. Cut the pork belly with scissors into 1-inch rectangular pieces.
20. Repeat steps 16-19 for the remaining batch of pork belly.
21. Set up the table family style for everyone to enjoy the short ribs and the pork belly.
22. Serve immediately and pair with lettuce for wrapping, sesame oil and sea salt for dipping the pork belly, ssamjang and green onion slices for lettuce wraps, and white rice if desired.

Marinated Steak and Veggie Kebabs

Cooking Time: 8 minutes   Servings: 5

INGREDIENTS

√ ¼ cup Worcestershire sauce
√ ¼ cup soy sauce
√ ¼ cup olive oil
√ 2 teaspoons Dijon mustard
√ 1 tablespoon minced garlic
√ ½ tablespoon brown sugar
√ 2 tablespoons lemon juice
√ 1 teaspoon hot sauce
√ 1 teaspoon black pepper
√ 1 pound beef tri-tip, cut into 1-inch cubes
√ 2 red bell peppers, cut into 1-inch pieces
√ 1 red onion, cut into 1-inch pieces

DIRECTIONS

1. Combine the Worcestershire sauce, soy sauce, olive oil, mustard, garlic, brown sugar, lemon juice, hot sauce, and pepper in a large bowl and whisk to combine.

2. Add the tri tip cubes into the bowl and evenly coat in the marinade. Cover the bowl with plastic wrap and place in the refrigerator for 4 hours.

3. Remove the bowl from the refrigerator, add the bell pepper and red onion, and toss to coat.

4. Select the Preheat function on the Cosori Air Fryer and press Start/Pause.

5. Skewer alternating pieces of steak and veggies until all the steak is used.

6. Insert the kebabs into the preheated air fryer.

7. Set temperature to 400°F and time to 8 minutes, then press Start/Pause.

8. Flip the kebabs halfway through cooking.

9. Remove the kebabs when done and let rest for 5 minutes before serving.

Chipotle Tuna Melt

Cooking Time: 13 minutes   Servings: 2

INGREDIENTS

√ 1 can (5 ounces) tuna
√ 3 tablespoons La Costeña Chipotle Sauce
√ 4 slices white bread
√ 2 slices pepper jack cheese

DIRECTIONS

1. SELECT Preheat on the Cosori Air Fryer, adjust to 320°F, and press Start/Pause.

2. MIX the tuna and chipotle sauce until combined.

3. SPREAD half of the chipotle tuna mixture onto each of 2 bread slices.

4. ADD a slice of pepper jack cheese onto each and top with the remaining 2 bread slices, making 2 sandwiches.

5. PLACE the sandwiches into the preheated air fryer.

6. SELECT Bread, adjust time to 8 minutes, and press Start/Pause.

7. CUT diagonally and serve.

Garam Masala & Yogurt-Marinated Cornish Game Hens

Cooking Time: 20 minutes   Servings: 2

INGREDIENTS
√ 1 Cornish hen
√ ¾ cup Greek yogurt
√ 3 limes, zested and juiced
√ 4 garlic cloves, grated
√ 2" piece fresh ginger, peeled and grated
√ 4 tablespoons olive oil
√ 3 tablespoons garam masala
√ 2 tablespoons ground turmeric
√ 2 tablespoons kosher salt
√ 1 teaspoon freshly ground black pepper
√ ½ teaspoon ground coriander
√ Oil spray

DIRECTIONS
1. Cut the hen down the spine using a pair of poultry shears and press the breast bone so they lay flat, then flip over and cut down the breast bone so the hens are halved down the center. Pat them very dry with paper towels.

2. Combine all of the ingredients except for the hen halves in a medium bowl and whisk well. Reserve half of the mixture in a separate bowl to use as a dipping sauce. Add the hen halves to the remaining mixture and spread to cover with the marinade. Cover and refrigerate for 2 and a half hours.

3. Remove the hens from the refrigerator and allow to come to room temperature 30 minutes prior to grilling.

4. Place the cooking pot into the base of the Cosori Indoor Grill, followed by the grill grate.

5. Select the Air Grill function on medium heat, adjust time to 20 minutes, press Shake, then press Start/Pause to preheat.

6. Spray the grill grate with oil spray, then place the Cornish hen halves onto the preheated grill grate skin side down and close the lid to begin cooking.

7. Flip chicken over halfway through cooking. The Shake reminder will let you know when.

8. Remove the Cornish hens and allow them to rest for 5-10 minutes before serving with the reserved yogurt sauce on the side.

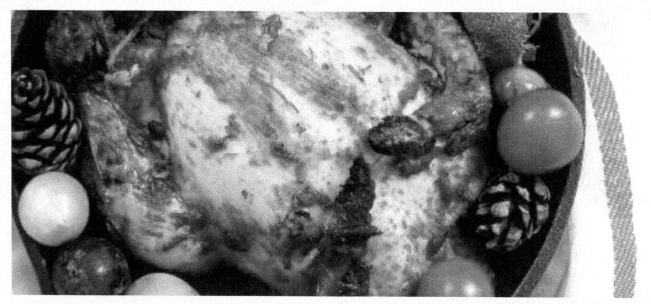

SoCal Veggie Grilled Cheese

Cooking Time: 9 minutes   Servings: 2

INGREDIENTS

√ 2 tablespoons mayonnaise
√ 4 slices crusty Italian bread, about ½-inch-thick
√ 1½ tablespoons crème fraîche
√ ½ zucchini, thinly sliced lengthwise
√ 1 clove garlic, thinly sliced
√ 2 teaspoons olive oil, divided
√ ½ teaspoon freshly ground black pepper, divided
√ 1 teaspoon kosher salt, divided
√ 6 ounces Havarti, sliced
√ 6 ounces provolone, sliced
√ 1 cup arugula
√ 2 tablespoons fresh basil leaves, torn
√ 1 tablespoon fresh dill, torn

DIRECTIONS

1. Spread the mayonnaise on both sides of each slice of bread, then spread the crème fraîche on the inside of 2 slices.

2. Layer the zucchini and garlic over the slices with the crème fraîche. Drizzle 1 tablespoon of the olive oil over the zucchini on each slice, then season each slice evenly with ¼ teaspoon pepper and ½ teaspoon salt.

3. Layer the Havarti and provolone cheese on the other 2 slices of bread, then combine with the slices layered with zucchini to form 2 sandwiches.

4. Place the cooking pot into the base of the Cosori Indoor Grill, followed by the basket.

5. Place the sandwiches into the preheated basket, then close the lid.

6. Select the Broil function, adjust time to 6 minutes, and press the Preheat button to bypass preheating. Press Start/Pause to begin cooking.

7. Open the lid and flip the sandwiches.

8. Select the Broil function, adjust time 3 minutes, then press Start/Pause.

9. Remove the sandwiches when done.

10. Toss the arugula, basil, and dill with the remaining olive oil, salt, and pepper, then divide the mixture between the 2 sandwiches.

11. Serve the sandwiches immediately.

Char Siu Dinner

INGREDIENTS

Marinade:
√ 1 teaspoon five-spice powder
√ 2 teaspoons kosher salt
√ ¼ teaspoon ground white pepper
√ 4 tablespoons granulated sugar
√ 1½ tablespoons soy sauce
√ 2 tablespoons hoisin sauce
√ 1 tablespoon Chinese rice wine
√ 2 tablespoons honey
√ 2 garlic cloves, minced
√ 2 cubes red fermented bean curd, mashed
√ 3 teaspoons red fermented bean curd liquid

Pork:
√ 2 pounds Boston butt (pork shoulder), tops and sides scored
√ 3 tablespoons honey
√ Oil spray

For Serving:
√ 2 cups short grain white rice, steamed
√ 1 cup Taiwanese cabbage, sauteed, for serving
√ Items Needed:
√ Pastry brush

DIRECTIONS

1. Combine marinade ingredients in a large bowl and mix until well combined. Set 4 tablespoons of marinade aside in the refrigerator.

2. Remove the thick, fatty pork rinds from around the entire piece of pork shoulder.

3. Slice the pork into smaller pieces, about 2-cm long and ¾-inch thick.

4. Place the pork and marinade into a large resealable plastic bag and shake until fully coated. Marinate for 1-2 days in the refrigerator.

5. Rest the pork for 30 minutes at room temperature before cooking.

6. Select the Preheat function on the Cosori Air Fryer, adjust temperature to 400°F, and press Start/Pause.

7. Mix the honey, 1½ tablespoons of water, and the 4 tablespoons of reserved marinade in a small bowl to make a basting mixture.

8. Spray the inner basket of the air fryer with oil spray.

9. Brush both sides of the pork slices with the basting mixture, then place into the preheated air fryer.

Note: The pieces pork can be touching each other, but should not be stacked on top of each other. You may need to work in batches.

10. Set temperature to 400°F and time to 12 minutes, press Shake, then press Start/Pause.

11. Flip the pork pieces over and brush more of the basting mixture on each side halfway through cooking. The Shake Reminder will let you know when.

12. Remove the pork when done, then transfer to a wire rack.

13. Baste the top of the pork with the remaining basting mixture.

14. Serve the Char Siu over steamed white rice with a side of sautéed Taiwanese cabbage.

Sweet Potato & Cranberry Stuffing Stuffed Turkey

Cooking Time: 45 minutes   Servings: 6

INGREDIENTS

√ 1 yellow onion, medium diced
√ 2 tablespoons unsalted butter
√ 1 medium sweet potato, ½-inch cubes
√ 1 stem celery, medium diced
√ 2 garlic cloves, minced
√ 1½ cups chicken broth, divided
√ Items Needed:
√ Butcher's twine
√ 2 tablespoons sage, rough chopped
√ 5 cups store-bought sourdough stuffing
√ ¼ teaspoon kosher salt
√ ¼ teaspoon ground black pepper
√ 3 boneless, skinless turkey breasts (1 pound each)

DIRECTIONS

1. Sauté the onions in butter in a saucepan over medium-high heat until translucent, about 2 minutes. Add in the sweet potato, celery, and garlic and cook for another 5 minutes.

2. Add 1 cup of chicken broth to the saucepan and bring the mixture to a boil.

3. Cover the pot and let the mixture boil for 7 minutes.

4. Add the remaining ½ cup of chicken broth, cranberries, and sage, then bring the mixture back to a boil.

5. Add in the stuffing and stir until fully combined. Continue cooking on high heat until the stuffing absorbs all the liquid.

6. Cover the pot, remove from heat, and set aside.

7. Combine the salt and pepper in a small bowl.

8. Butterfly the turkey breasts to yield a ½-inch-thick larger turkey breast.

9. Season the turkey breasts with the salt and pepper mixture on both sides.

10. Divide the stuffing mixture into 3 equal portions.

11. Place the stuffing mixture onto the bottom of each butterflied turkey breast.

12. Roll the turkey breasts up, starting from the bottom. After each roll is made, make sure to tuck and tighten the sides to keep the stuffing secure.

13. Secure the roulades by using butcher's twine, and place into the Cosori Air Fryer baskets.

14. Select the Bake function, adjust time to 45 minutes, then press Start/Pause.

15. Remove the turkey roulades from the air fryer when done.

16. Cover the turkey roulades with foil and let rest for 8 minutes.

17. Slice into ½-inch-thick slices to create 5 slices per roulade.

18. Serve immediately.

Citrus & Herb Turkey Breast

Cooking Time: 40 minutes   Servings: 4

INGREDIENTS

√ 1 teaspoon aniseed or fennel seed
√ 4 teaspoons kosher salt
√ 2 teaspoons orange zest, finely grated
√ 1 teaspoon dark brown sugar
√ 2 teaspoons fresh rosemary leaves, roughly chopped

Items Needed:

√ Spice grinder or mortar and pestle
√ Food processor
√ 2 teaspoons fresh thyme leaves
√ ½ teaspoon freshly ground black pepper
√ 1 turkey half-breast with rib meat (2.5 pounds)
√ 4 teaspoons olive oil
√ Rimmed baking sheet

DIRECTIONS

1. Toast the aniseed or fennel seed in a small, dry skillet over medium heat, stirring occasionally, for about 2 minutes, or until fragrant and lightly toasted. Set aside to cool.

2. Grind the aniseed or fennel seed finely in a spice grinder or using a mortar and pestle.

3. Place the salt, orange zest, brown sugar, rosemary, thyme, pepper, and aniseed (or fennel seed) in a food processor.

4. Pulse until herbs are finely chopped.

5. Rub the herb mixture all over the turkey breast, then place on a rimmed baking sheet.

6. Chill in the refrigerator uncovered for 4-6 hours.

7. Rinse the turkey breast, pat very dry, and place back on the baking sheet, skin-side up. Allow the turkey breast to sit at room temperature while you preheat the air fryer.

8. Select the Preheat function on the Cosori Air Fryer, adjust temperature to 330°F, and press Start/Pause.

9. Rub the olive oil all over the turkey breast.

10. Place the turkey breast skin-side up into the preheated air fryer basket.

11. Adjust temperature to 330°F and time to 40 minutes, then press Start/Pause.

12. Remove the turkey breast when golden brown and fully cooked.

13. Rest the turkey for 10 minutes, then slice and serve.

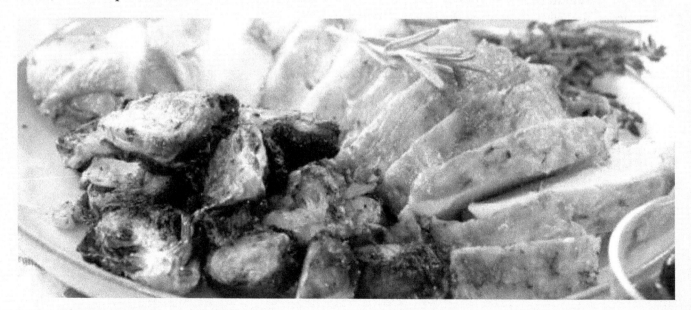

Honey and Soy Marinated Salmon

Cooking Time: 8 minutes   Servings: 2

INGREDIENTS

√ 1 tablespoon grapeseed oil
√ 1 tablespoon honey
√ 1 garlic clove, minced
√ ¼ teaspoon salt
√ 2 salmon fillets (4 ounces each)
√ ½ teaspoon white sesame seeds, toasted, for garnish
√ White rice, for serving

Items Needed:

√ Sheet pan
√ ¼ teaspoon sesame oil
√ 1 tablespoon soy sauce (or liquid aminos)
√ 1 tablespoon green onion, chopped, plus more for garnish
√ ⅛ teaspoon ground white pepper
√ Oil spray
√ Chinese broccoli or Bok Choy, for serving

DIRECTIONS

1. Whisk together the grapeseed oil, sesame oil, honey, soy sauce, garlic, onion, salt, and pepper in a bowl to make the marinade.
2. Reserve 1 tablespoon of the marinade for later use.
3. Add the salmon and marinade to a resealable freezer bag and seal. Shake to coat the salmon with the marinade.
4. Marinate the salmon in the refrigerator for 30 minutes.
5. Select the Preheat function on the Cosori Air Fryer, adjust temperature to 350°F, then press Start/Pause.
6. Spray the inner air fryer basket with oil spray.
7. Remove salmon from the marinade and place in the preheated air fryer baskets.
8. Select the Seafood function, then press Start/Pause.
9. Remove the salmon when done and transfer onto a sheet pan lined with parchment paper.
10. Allow the salmon to rest for 3 minutes before serving. Garnish with white sesame seeds and green onions.
11. Serve with white rice and Chinese broccoli or Bok Choy.

45

Kale Salad with Crispy Chickpeas

Cooking Time: 12 minutes   Servings: 4

INGREDIENTS

For the Chickpeas:

√ One 15-ounce can chickpeas, drained, rinsed, & patted dry

√ 1 tablespoon olive oil

√ ½ teaspoon kosher salt

√ ¼ teaspoon black pepper

√ ¼ teaspoon garlic powder

√ ¼ teaspoon paprika

√ ¼ teaspoon cumin

√ ¼ teaspoon coriander

√ ⅛ teaspoon cayenne pepper

For the Salad:

√ 1 large bunch of kale

√ 1 tablespoon olive oil

√ 1 tablespoon lemon juice

√ For the Dressing:

√ 2 cloves garlic, minced

√ 1/3 cup tahini

√ 2 tablespoons olive oil

√ ¼ cup lemon juice

√ 1 tablespoon maple syrup

√ 1 tablespoon hot water

√ ½ teaspoon salt

√ ¼ teaspoon black pepper

DIRECTIONS

1. Select the Preheat function on the Cosori Air Fryer and press Start/Pause.

2. Combine all the chickpea ingredients together in a bowl and toss to combine.

3. Place the chickpeas into the preheated air fryer basket.

4. Set temperature to 400°F and time to 12 minutes, press Shake, then press Start/Pause.

5. Shake the chickpeas halfway through cooking. The Shake Reminder will let you know when.

6. Remove the chickpeas when golden and crispy.

7. Combine all the dressing ingredients in a small bowl, then whisk until smooth. Adjust consistency by adding more hot water if too thick.

8. Prepare the salad by removing the ribs from the kale. Slice the kale leaves into ¾-inch-thick ribbons.

9. Place the kale in a large mixing bowl. Add the olive oil and lemon juice, then massage the kale with your hands to soften the texture and reduce the bitterness.

10. Add as much dressing as you like and toss to coat.

11. Top with the crispy chickpeas and serve.

Crispy Curry Chicken Tenders

Cooking Time: 480 minutes   Servings: 4

INGREDIENTS

√ 1 pound boneless skinless chicken tenders
√ ¼ cup plain yogurt
√ 2 tablespoons thai red curry paste
√ 1½ teaspoons salt, divided
√ ½ teaspoon pepper
√ 1¾ cups panko breadcrumbs
√ 1 teaspoon granulated garlic
√ 1 teaspoon granulated onion
√ Olive oil or avocado oil spray

DIRECTIONS

1. Whisk together the yogurt, curry paste, 1 teaspoon of salt, and pepper in a large bowl. Add the chicken tenders and toss to coat. Cover bowl with plastic wrap and marinate in the fridge for 6-8 hours.
2. Combine the panko breadcrumbs, ½ teaspoon salt, garlic, and onion. Remove chicken tenders from the marinade and coat individually in the panko mixture.
3. Select the Preheat function on the Cosori Smart Air Fryer Toaster Oven, adjust temperature to 430°F, and press Start/Pause.
4. Spray both sides of each chicken tender well with olive oil or avocado oil spray, then place into the fry basket.
5. Insert the fry basket at mid position in the preheated oven.
6. Select the Air Fry and Shake functions, adjust time to 14 minutes, and press Start/Pause.
7. Flip chicken tenders halfway through cooking. The Shake Reminder will let you know when.
8. Remove when chicken tenders are golden and crispy.

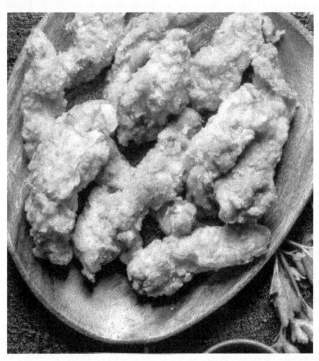

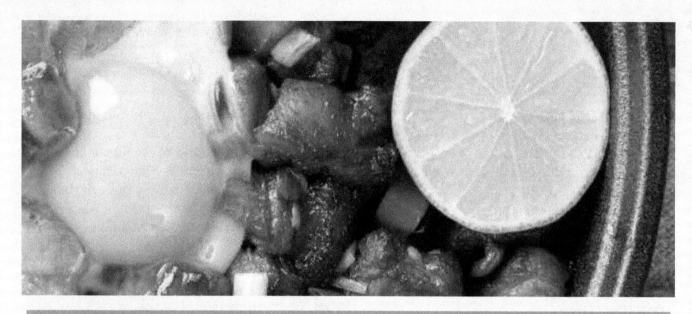

Pork Belly Sisig

Cooking Time: 25 minutes Servings: 4-5

INGREDIENTS

√ 2 pounds pork belly, cut into ½-inch thick cubes

√ 2¼ teaspoons garlic salt

√ 1 teaspoon freshly ground black pepper, plus more for sprinkling

√ 4 tablespoons freshly squeezed lemon or calamansi juice

√ 2 tablespoons low-sodium soy sauce

√ 3-4 red chili peppers, sliced

√ 5 scallions, chopped

√ 1 egg

DIRECTIONS

1. Season the pork belly with garlic salt and black pepper.

2. Select the Preheat function on the Cosori Air Fryer and press Start/Pause.

3. Place the pork belly cubes into the preheated air fryer basket.

4. Select the Steak function, set time to 10 minutes, and press Start/Pause.

5. Mix together lemon juice and soy sauce into a large bowl.

6. Place the cooked pork belly into the lemon soy mixture along with sliced chilis and chopped scallions. Toss the ingredients together and set aside.

7. Pour 1 tablespoon of the fat dripping from the pork belly in the cake pan accessory.

8. Place the pan into a clean air fryer basket.

9. Select the Preheat function, adjust to 350°F, and press Start/Pause.

10. Add the pork belly, scallions, chiles, and sauce to the cake pan accessory. Then crack an egg on top.

11. Adjust the temperature to 350°F, set time for 5 minutes, and press Start/Pause.

12. Serve with a side of lemon or calamansi and chilis.

Lobster Rolls

INGREDIENTS

√ ¼ teaspoon dried oregano

√ ¼ teaspoon dried thyme

√ ¼ teaspoon celery salt

√ ¼ teaspoon freshly ground black pepper

√ 4 (3-ounce) lobster tails

√ Ice water bath

√ 3 tablespoons mayonnaise

√ 2 teaspoons freshly chopped tarragon

√ 2 teaspoons freshly chopped chives

√ 1 tablespoon finely chopped celery

√ 1 tablespoon finely chopped shallots

√ Salt, to taste

√ 2 split top hot dog buns

√ Melted butter, for brushing

DIRECTIONS

1. Mix together the dried oregano, dried thyme, celery salt, and black pepper together and blend in a blender until it forms a fine powder. Set aside.

2. Select the Preheat function on the Cosori Air Fryer, adjust temperature to 370°F, then press Start/Pause.

3. Place lobster tails into the preheated air fryer basket with shell side up.

4. Select the Shrimp function, set time to 8 minutes, and press Start/Pause. Flip halfway through cooking.

5. Place the lobster in the ice bath for 5 minutes, remove from the shell, and cut into chunks.

6. Mix the mayonnaise, chopped tarragon, chopped chives, ½ teaspoon of the seasoning powder, chopped celery, and chopped shallots with the lobster until well combined.

7. Season the lobster to taste with salt and store in the fridge for at least 10 minutes.

8. Brush the buns on each side with the melted butter and toast the buns in the pan over medium heat until golden brown, about 3-5 minutes on each side.

9. Divide the lobster evenly between the buns and enjoy.

BBQ Tofu Kebabs

Cooking Time: 70 minutes   Servings: 5

INGREDIENTS

√ 15-ounce block firm tofu, pressed and cut into 1-inch cubes
√ 1 bell pepper, cut into 1-inch cubes
√ 1 red onion, cut into 1-inch cubes
√ 1 zucchini, cut into 1-inch pieces
√ 2 tablespoons bbq sauce
√ 2 tablespoons soy sauce
√ 1 tablespoons sriracha
√ 1 tablespoon maple syrup
√ 1 tablespoon olive oil
√ 2 tablespoons water
√ 2 garlic cloves, minced
√ 1 teaspoon black pepper

DIRECTIONS

1. Combine bbq sauce, soy sauce, sriracha, maple syrup, olive oil, water, garlic, and black pepper in a bowl and whisk together. Add tofu cubes and toss to coat. Place in the refrigerator to marinate for 1 hour. Remove tofu from the refrigerator.
2. Skewer alternating pieces of tofu and veggies until all the tofu is used.
3. Select the Preheat function on the Cosori Air Fryer, and press Start/Pause.
4. Insert kebabs into the preheated air fryer basket. Brush the tops of the kebabs with marinade.
5. Set the temperature to 400°F, time to 10 minutes, and press Start/Pause. Flip halfway through cooking and brush the tops with more marinade.
6. Remove kebabs and serve.

BBQ Dry Rubbed Chicken Wings

Cooking Time: 35 minutes   Servings: 3-4

INGREDIENTS

√ 2 teaspoons chili powder
√ 1 teaspoon light brown sugar, packed
√ ½ teaspoon kosher salt
√ ½ teaspoon smoked paprika
√ ½ teaspoon ground paprika
√ ½ teaspoon onion powder
√ 1/3 teaspoon ground cumin
√ ¼ teaspoon garlic powder
√ ¼ teaspoon cayenne pepper
√ ¼ teaspoon ground mustard
√ A pinch of freshly ground black pepper
√ A pinch of dried oregano
√ A pinch of dried thyme
√ A pinch of dried rosemary
√ 2 pounds chicken wings
√ 2 tablespoons apple cider vinegar
√ 1 tablespoon canola oil

DIRECTIONS

1. Combine all the dried seasoning ingredients and mix well.
2. Sprinkle the dried seasoning all over the chicken wings.
3. Mix in apple cider vinegar and canola oil until all the wings are coated and wet.
4. Select the Preheat function on the Cosori Air Fryer, adjust to 380°F, and press Start/Pause.
5. Place the seasoned wings in the preheated air fryer basket.
6. Select the Chicken function and press Start/Pause.

Lemon & Dill Chicken Salad

Cooking Time: 273 minutes   Servings: 2-3

INGREDIENTS

√ 1 pound chicken tenderloins
√ 4 tablespoons extra-virgin olive oil, divided
√ 3 tablespoons lemon juice, divided
√ 1½ tablespoon dijon mustard, divided
√ 4 teaspoons freshly chopped dill, divided
√ 2 garlic cloves, grated
√ ¼ teaspoon onion powder
√ ¼ teaspoon garlic powder
√ Sea salt and freshly ground black pepper, to taste
√ 1 tablespoon apple cider vinegar
√ 1 lemon, zested
√ 1 small sweet potato, peeled and cut into ½ X 3-inch strips
√ 4 cups baby spinach
√ 8 ounces cherry tomatoes, halved
√ 1 medium cucumber, sliced
√ 1 large avocado, halved and sliced
√ Fresh dill, for garnish
√ Fresh italian parsley, for garnish

DIRECTIONS

1. Place the chicken tenders in a Ziploc bag.
2. Mix together 1 tablespoon extra-virgin olive oil, 2 tablespoons lemon juice, 1 tablespoon dijon mustard, 2 teaspoons freshly chopped dill, grated garlic, and onion powder to make the marinade.
3. Season the marinade with salt and pepper to taste.
4. Pour the marinade into the bag of chicken and marinate in the fridge for 4 hours.
5. Whisk together 3 tablespoons extra virgin olive oil, 1 tablespoon lemon juice, ½ tablespoon dijon mustard, 2 teaspoons of freshly chopped dill, apple cider vinegar, and lemon zest until it forms a homogeneous vinaigrette. Then season to taste with salt and pepper and set aside.
6. Select the Preheat function on the Cosori Air Frye and press Start/Pause.
7. Remove the chicken from the fridge and marinade, then place it into the preheated air fryer basket.
8. Adjust the temperature to 400°F, set time to 8 minutes, and press Start/Pause.
9. Remove the chicken from the air fryer and allow it to rest for 10 minutes before slicing into pieces.
10. Drizzle the sweet potatoes with the leftover marinade and place into the air fryer basket.
11. Adjust the temperature to 400°F, set time to 10 minutes, and press Start/Pause.
12. Toss together the baby spinach, halved cherry tomatoes, sliced cucumber, sliced avocado, sliced chicken, and roasted sweet potatoes in a large bowl until well combined.
13. Pour the ¾ of the vinaigrette on the sides of the bowl and toss until the ingredients are evenly coated. (you can add more of the vinaigrette if you like)
14. Garnish with fresh dill and fresh Italian parsley.

Supreme French Bread Pizza

Cooking Time: 28 minutes   Servings: 4-5

INGREDIENTS

√ 1 loaf French bread, 4-inches X 14-inches
√ 3 tablespoons salted butter
√ 3 tablespoons extra-virgin olive oil, divided
√ 4 cloves garlic, finely minced
√ ½ teaspoon dried oregano
√ A pinch red pepper flakes
√ ½ cup marinara sauce
√ 8 ounces shredded mozzarella cheese
√ 2 ounces grated Parmigiano-reggiano
√ Cooked ground italian sausage
√ Pepperoni slices
√ ¼ cup chopped red onion
√ ¼ cup chopped green bell pepper
√ ¼ cup chopped red bell pepper
√ Kosher salt, for sprinkling
√ Freshly ground black pepper, for sprinkling

DIRECTIONS

1. Half the french bread lengthwise, then crosswise.
2. Press the bread down until it is about 2/3 the original thickness and set aside.
3. Mix together butter, olive oil, garlic, dried oregano, red pepper flakes in a sauce pot and heat over medium heat until butter is fully melted.
4. Brush both sides of the bread slices with the garlic butter mixture.
5. Select the Preheat function on the Cosori Air Fryer, adjust the temperature to 320°F, and press Start/Pause.
6. Place the buttered bread in the preheated air fryer basket. You may need to work in batches.
7. Select the Bread function and press Start/Pause.
8. Remove the bread and spread a layer of marinara sauce on the open side of the loaf.
9. Mix together the cheese mixture and sprinkle on top of the marinara sauce.
10. Top the cheese with ground italian sausage, pepperoni, red onion, green bell peppers, and red bell peppers.
11. Sprinkle the tops with salt and black pepper.
12. Select the Preheat function on the Cosori Air Fryer, adjust the temperature to 350°F, and press Start/Pause.
13. Place the pizzas in the preheated air fryer basket. You may need to work in batches.
14. Adjust temperature to 350°F, set time for 4 minutes, and press Start/Pause.

Stuffed Jack O Lanterns

INGREDIENTS

√ 2 tablespoons olive oil, divided
√ 8 ounces spicy Italian sausage, ground
√ ½ white onion, diced
√ 2 Roma tomatoes, diced
√ 1 clove garlic, minced
√ 1 cup rice, cooked
√ 2 orange bell peppers

DIRECTIONS

1. Heat 1 tablespoon oil in a skillet over medium heat.

2. Cook the Italian sausage in the skillet until brown. Set aside.

3. Heat 1 tablespoon oil in the same skillet.

4. Add diced onion and cook for 5 minutes.

5. Add diced tomatoes and minced garlic. Cook for another 5 minutes, then set aside.

6. Mix sausage, onions, tomatoes, garlic, and cooked rice together, then set aside.

7. Cut off the tops of the bell peppers. Leave the stems on the tops and remove the seeds and ribs from the body of the peppers.

8. Cut jack-o-lantern faces in the bell peppers.

9. Select the Preheat function on the Cosori Air Fryer, set temperature to 320°F, then press Start/Pause.

10. Stuff the peppers with the sausage and rice mix.

11. Place the peppers along with the tops into the preheated air fryer.

12. Set the time to 5 minutes, then press Start/Pause.

13. Remove when done and serve immediately.

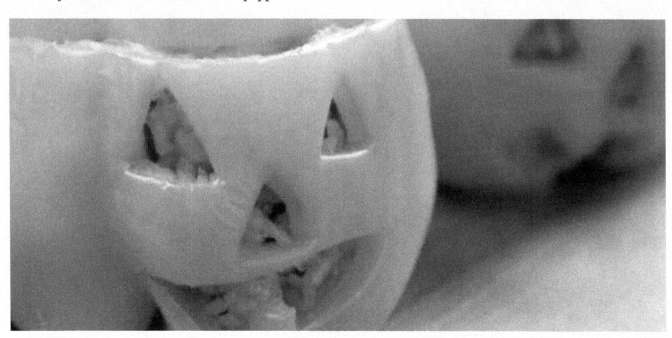

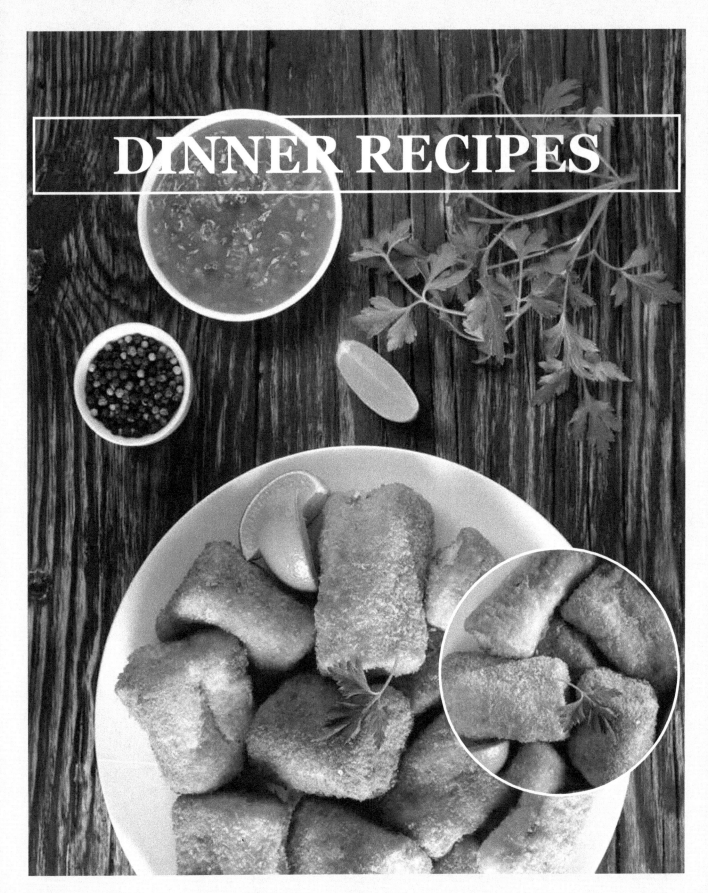

DINNER RECIPES

Crispy Fried Chicken

INGREDIENTS

√ 6 pieces bone in, skin on chicken - cut of your choice

√ 3 tablespoons kosher salt, divided, plus more for sprinkling

√ 2 cups buttermilk

√ 2 oz vodka

√ 1 whole egg + 1 egg white

√ 2 bay leaf

√ Several fresh thyme sprigs

√ 1 tablespoon hot sauce

√ 1 cup all purpose flour

√ 1 cup cornstarch

√ 1 teaspoon baking powder

√ 1/2 tablespoon paprika

√ 1/2 teaspoon cayenne pepper

√ 1/2 tablespoon dried oregano

√ 1/2 tablespoon garlic powder

√ 1/2 tablespoon dried thyme leaves

√ 1/2 tablespoon onion powder

√ 1/2 tablespoon black pepper

√ 1/2 teaspoon chili powder

DIRECTIONS

1. Set chicken on a plate or rimmed baking sheet, skin side up, and sprinkle with kosher salt. Let sit for 30 minutes in the refrigerator before beginning the marinade process.

2. Combine buttermilk, vodka, 2 tbsp kosher salt, pepper, bay leaves, egg, thyme and hot sauce in a large bowl. Submerge chicken pieces and allow to marinate in the refrigerator for at least two hours or up to overnight.

3. Combine flour, cornstarch, paprika, cayenne, oregano, dried thyme, garlic powder, onion powder, chili powder, 1 tbsp kosher salt, and black pepper in a bowl. Whisk to combine.

4. Remove chicken from the buttermilk marinade and shake to remove excess. Dredge the chicken in the flour mixture and set each one on a rimmed baking sheet fitted with a wire rack. Let the chicken rest, battered, for 30 minutes before frying.

5. Preheat the Cosori Air Fryer to 380 degrees for 5 minutes.

6. Place the chicken in a single layer, skin side down, in the air fryer upper basket (you may need to work in batches). Close the drawer, and cook for 12 minutes at 380 degrees. When the timer goes off, spray any parts that are still floury looking with grapeseed or canola oil. Flip the chicken over and then cook for an additional 10 minutes at 380 degrees. Test the thickest part of the chicken with a thermometer, being careful not to touch the bone with the tip of the thermometer. The internal temperature should be between 160 and 165 degrees.

7. Allow chicken to rest for 5 minutes before serving.

Dry-Rubbed Steak

Cooking Time: 6 minutes   Servings: 1-2

INGREDIENTS
√ 1 ribeye (or NY) steak, 1-inch thick, room temperature
√ 1 tablespoon kosher salt
√ 1 tablespoon dark brown sugar, packed
√ 2 teaspoons paprika
√ 2 teaspoons ancho chile pepper
√ 1 teaspoon black pepper
√ ½ teaspoon garlic powder
√ ½ teaspoon onion powder
√ ½ teaspoon mustard powder
√ ½ teaspoon ground cumin
√ 1 teaspoon dried oregano

DIRECTIONS
1. Combine salt, brown sugar, paprika, ancho chile pepper, black pepper, garlic powder, onion powder, mustard powder, cumin, and dried oregano.
2. Dry steak thoroughly with paper towels.
3. Rub the spice mixture generously over the steak and allow to sit at room temperature for 20 minutes.
4. Preheat the air fryer to 400°F.
5. Place the steak in the preheated air fryer.
6. Cook at 400°F for 6 minutes.
7. Allow the steak to rest for 10 minutes before slicing.

Slow Roasted Lemon Garlic Chicken

Cooking Time: 125 minutes   Servings: 4

INGREDIENTS
√ 1 5-pound whole chicken
√ 2 tablespoons olive oil
√ 2 tablespoons kosher salt
√ 1 ½ teaspoons lemon pepper
√ 1 teaspoon garlic powder
√ 1 lemon, quartered
√ 1 garlic bulb, cut in half lengthwise
√ 1 sprig rosemary
√ ¾ cup white wine

DIRECTIONS
1. Pat the chicken dry and remove the insides. Drizzle olive oil over and massage into the chicken. Season all over and the inside cavity with salt, lemon pepper, and garlic powder.
2. Place the chicken in a deep baking dish that fits inside the air fryer oven. Place the quartered lemon, garlic bulb, and rosemary in the cavity of the chicken. Add the white wine in the bottom of the baking dish. Cover tightly with foil.
3. Place the baking dish onto the bottom rack of the air fryer oven.
4. Select the Slow Cook function, adjust time to 1 hour 45 minutes, and press Start/Pause.
5. Remove chicken when the internal temperature reaches 160°F. Remove the foil.
6. Place the baking dish back into the air fryer oven. Select the Broil function, and press Start/Pause.
7. Remove when chicken is golden and skin is crispy.
8. Allow chicken to rest for 15 minutes before carving and serving.

Fried Chicken

Cooking Time: 45 minutes   Servings: 4

INGREDIENTS

√ 3 eggs
√ ½ cup buffalo wing sauce
√ 4 chicken legs
√ 4 chicken thighs
√ 1½ cup all-purpose flour
√ 1/3 cup cornstarch
√ 2 teaspoons kosher salt
√ 2 teaspoons ground paprika
√ 1 teaspoon ground mustard
√ 1 teaspoon garlic powder
√ 1 teaspoon onion powder
√ ½ teaspoon ground ginger
√ ½ teaspoon dried oregano
√ ½ teaspoon dried thyme
√ ½ teaspoon dried basil
√ ½ teaspoon black pepper
√ ½ teaspoon ground white pepper
√ ½ teaspoon cayenne pepper
√ Cooking spray

DIRECTIONS

1. Whisk together eggs and buffalo wing sauce until well combined.

2. Marinate the chicken in the egg and buffalo wing sauce mixture for 30 minutes.

3. Whisk together the flour, cornstarch, and seasonings until well combined.

4. Drizzle 2 tablespoons of the marinade into the seasoned flour and use your hands to create small crumbs.

5. Dredge the chicken in the seasoned flour pressing down the flour into the chicken until it is fully covered.

6. Remove the clumped flour off your hands and mix back into the flour. This will create a crispier breading.

7. Spray the chicken liberally with cooking spray on both sides and arrange the chicken on the air fryer basket. Set aside.

8. Select the Air Fry and Preheat functions, adjust to 360F, set time to 30 minutes, and press Start/ Pause.

9. Place the chicken onto the middle rack of the preheated air fryer oven, then press Start/Pause. The air fryer oven will let you know when it is done preheating.

10. Remove the chicken when done cooking and allow to cool for 10 minutes before serving.

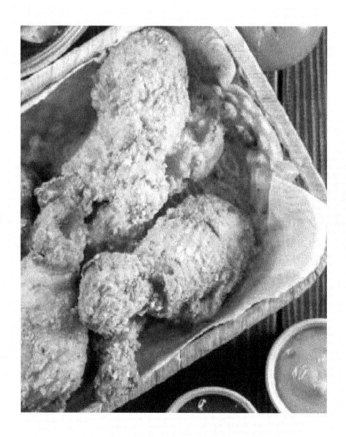

Mushroom Pizza

Cooking Time: 218 minutes   Servings: 6

INGREDIENTS
Dough
√ 1¼ cup all-purpose flour
√ ½ teaspoon kosher salt
√ ½ cup warm water (100-110°F)
√ 1 teaspoon honey
√ ½ teaspoon instant dry yeast
√ ½ teaspoon olive oil, plus more for drizzling
Toppings
√ ½ cup pizza sauce
√ 3 ounces low moisture mozzarella cheese, shredded
√ 5 ounces mushrooms, sliced
√ 1 roma tomato, diced
√ 2 tablespoons freshly chopped basil
√ Kosher salt and freshly ground black pepper, to taste

DIRECTIONS
1. Mix together flour and salt until well combined in a bowl. Set aside.
2. Whisk together water, honey, yeast, and olive oil in a large bowl. Allow the yeast to bloom for 5 minutes.
3. Mix in the flour into the bloomed yeast, mix until just combined, then cover and allow the dough to rest for 30 minutes.
4. Place the dough onto a lightly floured surface and knead until it forms a ball, about 3 minutes.
5. Place the dough on a lightly floured surface and dust the top of the dough lightly with flour as well.
6. Cover the dough with plastic wrap and rest in a warm place for 2 hours or until doubled in size.
7. Drizzle olive oil onto the food tray and rub along the sides of the pan.
8. Stretch the rested dough and place onto the oiled food tray.

9. Drizzle some olive oil on top of the dough and rub it on the top.
10. Cover the dough and allow it to rest for 1 hour.
11. Stretch the dough to fill out the sides of the food tray.
12. Spread the top of the dough with pizza sauce, followed by mozzarella cheese, then mushrooms, mushrooms, and chopped basil.
13. Sprinkle the top of the pizza to taste with salt and freshly ground black pepper.
14. Select the Pizza and Preheat functions on the Cosori Air Fryer Oven, then press Start/Pause.
15. Place the pizza onto the middle rack of the preheated air fryer oven, then press Start/Pause. The air fryer oven will let you know when it is done preheating.
16. Remove the pizza from the oven when done cooking and allow it to rest for 10 minutes.
17. Cut the pizza in slices and serve.

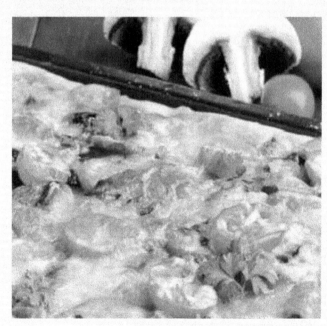

Korean "Fried" Chicken Wings

Cooking Time: 35 minutes   Servings: 4

INGREDIENTS

Wing

√ 2 pounds chicken wings
√ 1 teaspoon kosher salt
√ ½ teaspoon black pepper
√ 1½ teaspoons onion powder
√ 1½ teaspoons garlic powder
√ ¾ teaspoons ground mustard
√ 1 teaspoon gochugaru
√ 2 tablespoons cornstarch
√ 1 tablespoon water
√ Cooking spray
√ Toasted sesame seeds, for sprinkling

Sauce

√ 3 tablespoons Korean gojuchang red pepper paste
√ 2 tablespoon white distilled vinegar
√ 1 tablespoon hot water
√ 2 tablespoons honey
√ 1 tablespoon soy sauce

DIRECTIONS

1. Combine all the ingredients for the wings except the cooking spray and sesame seeds in a large bowl. Mix well.

2. Select the Preheat function on the Cosori Smart Air Fryer Toaster Oven, adjust temperature to 400°F, and press Start/Pause.

3. Spray both sides of the wings with cooking spray.

4. Place the wings into the fry basket, then insert the basket at mid position in the preheated oven.

5. Select the Air Fry function, adjust time to 25 minutes, then press Start/Pause.

6. Mix together sauce ingredients until well combined, then microwave on high for 30 seconds. Set aside.

7. Remove wings when done, then place the wings and sauce in a large bowl and toss together until the wings are well coated.

8. Sprinkle the wings with toasted sesame seeds and serve.

Mozzarella Stuffed Arancini

INGREDIENTS

√ 3½ cups low sodium chicken stock
√ 4 tablespoons unsalted butter, divided
√ 1 medium onion, finely chopped
√ 2 garlic cloves, minced
√ 1 cup arborio rice
√ 1½ teaspoons kosher salt, plus more to taste
√ ½ cup dry white wine
√ 2 ounces finely grated Parmesan
√ ¼ cup heavy cream
√ 1 teaspoon freshly ground black pepper, plus more to taste
√ 3 ounces low-moisture mozzarella, cut into 1/3-inch pieces
√ 1½ cups panko breadcrumbs
√ 2 tablespoons melted salted butter
√ ½ cup all-purpose flour
√ 2 large eggs, beaten
√ Cooking spray
√ Marinara sauce, for serving

DIRECTIONS

1. Simmer chicken stock in a pot, then keep warm on low heat.
2. Heat 2 tablespoons of unsalted butter in a medium saucepan over medium heat.
3. Add onions to the saucepan and cook for 5 minutes or until softened.
4. Add garlic and cook for 1 minute or until softened.
5. Add rice and 1½ teaspoons of kosher salt to the saucepan.
6. Cook the rice for 3 minutes or until the edges turn translucent.
7. Pour in the wine, stir, and cook for 3 minutes or until the wine is all evaporated and the rice looks dry.
8. Ladle in 1 cup of the warm chicken stock and bring to a simmer. Stirring often, cook the rice for 5 minutes or until liquid is absorbed. Repeat this process with another cup of chicken stock.
9. Add the remaining 1½ cups of chicken stock and cook, stirring often, for 10 minutes or until the rice is cooked through but toothsome and the liquid is mostly absorbed.
10. Remove the risotto from the heat and mix in Parmesan, heavy cream, black pepper, and the remaining two tablespoons of unsalted butter.
11. Season the risotto to taste with salt and black pepper.
12. Spread risotto in an even layer on a parchment-lined baking sheet and cover with plastic wrap.
13. Place the risotto in the fridge and chill for 4 hours.
14. Separate the chilled risotto into 14 even pieces and form them into round patties about 2½ inches in diameter.
15. Place a piece of mozzarella in the center of a patty, pinch and shape the risotto so it completely encases the cheese, then roll into a ball. Repeat with each risotto patty.
16. Place the balls onto the baking sheet lined with fresh parchment paper, cover with plastic wrap, and place in the freezer for 15 minutes.
17. Place the panko breadcrumbs into a food processor and pulse until finely ground, then place into a bowl.
18. Mix the panko breadcrumbs with the melted salted butter until well combined.
19. Remove the risotto balls from the freezer and dredge in flour, dip in beaten eggs, then cover with breadcrumbs. Repeat this process with the rest of the balls. Set aside.
20. Select the Preheat function on the Cosori Smart Air Fryer Toaster Oven, adjust temperature to 400°F, and press Start/Pause.
21. Place the balls into the fry basket, spray them liberally with cooking spray, then insert the basket at mid position in the preheated oven.
22. Select the Air Fry and Shake functions, adjust time to 20 minutes, and press Start/Pause.
23. Remove the arancini from the oven and serve with marinara sauce.

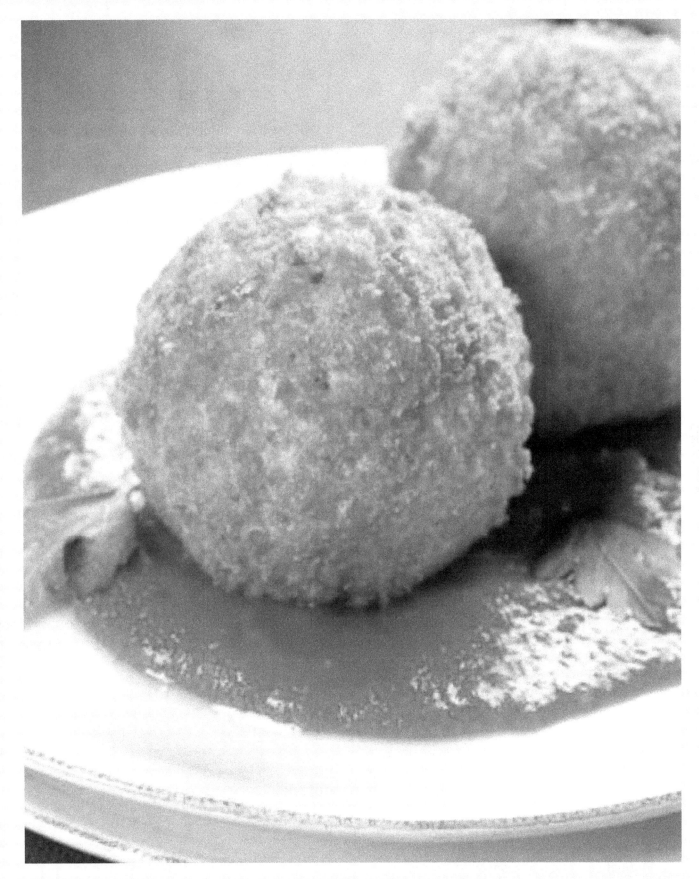

Ribeye Steak with Blue Cheese Compound Butter

Cooking Time: 262 minutes   Servings: 2

INGREDIENTS

√ 5 tablespoons unsalted butter, softened
√ ¼ cup crumbled blue cheese
√ 2 teaspoons lemon juice
√ 1 tablespoon freshly chopped chives
√ Salt & freshly ground black pepper, to taste
√ 2 (12 ounce) boneless ribeye steaks

DIRECTIONS

1. Mix together butter, blue cheese, lemon juice, and chives until smooth.
2. Season the butter to taste with salt and pepper.
3. Place the butter on plastic wrap and form into a 3-inch log, tying the ends of the plastic wrap together.
4. Place the butter in the fridge for 4 hours to harden.
5. Allow the steaks to sit at room temperature for 1 hour.
6. Pat the steaks dry with paper towels and season to taste with salt and pepper.
7. Insert the fry basket at top position in the Cosori Smart Air Fryer Toaster Oven.
8. Select the Preheat function, adjust temperature to 450°F, and press Start/Pause.
9. Place the steaks in the fry basket in the preheated oven.
10. Select the Broil function, adjust time to 12 minutes, and press Start/Pause.
11. Remove when done and allow to rest for 5 minutes.
12. Remove the butter from the fridge, unwrap, and slice into ¾-inch pieces.
13. Serve the steak with one or two pieces of sliced compound butter.

Harissa Lemon Whole Chicken

Cooking Time: 150 minutes   Servings: 6

INGREDIENTS

√ 2 teaspoons kosher salt
√ ½ teaspoon freshly ground black pepper
√ ½ teaspoon ground cumin
√ 2 garlic cloves
√ 6 tablespoons harissa paste
√ ½ lemon, juiced
√ 1 whole lemon, zested
√ 1 (5 pound) whole chicken

DIRECTIONS

1. Place salt, pepper, cumin, garlic cloves, harissa paste, lemon juice, and lemon zest in a food processor and pulse until they form a smooth puree.
2. Rub the puree all over the chicken, especially inside the cavity, and cover with plastic wrap.
3. Marinate for 1 hour at room temperature.
4. Select the Preheat function on the Cosori Smart Air Fryer Toaster Oven and press Start/Pause.
5. Place the marinated chicken on the food tray, then insert the tray at low position in the preheated oven.
6. Select the Roast function, then press Start/Pause.
7. Remove when done, tent chicken with foil, and allow it to rest for 20 minutes before serving.

Mahi Mahi Tacos with Pineapple Salsa

Cooking Time: 19 minutes   Servings: 2

INGREDIENTS

Salsa
√ 1 cup pineapple, diced
√ ½ lime, zested and juiced
√ 1 small jalapeno, diced
√ 1 avocado, diced
√ ¼ red onion, diced
√ 2 tablespoons cilantro, chopped
√ A pinch of salt

Mahi Mahi
√ 2 (6-ounce) filets of Mahi Mahi fish
√ 1 tablespoon olive oil
√ Salt & pepper, to taste
√ Corn tortillas for serving

DIRECTIONS

1. Combine all the salsa ingredients in a bowl. Stir together and taste, then add additional salt if desired. Store salsa in the fridge until ready to serve.

2. Select the Preheat function on the Cosori Smart Air Fryer Toaster Oven, adjust temperature to 430°F, and press Start/Pause.

3. Line the food tray with foil, then place mahi mahi on the tray. Drizzle with olive oil and season with salt and pepper.

4. Insert food tray at top position in the preheated oven.

5. Select the Air Fry function, adjust time to 9 minutes, and press Start/Pause.

6. Remove when the internal temperature of the mahi mahi reaches close to 145°F. Allow fish to rest for 5 minutes, then flake into large pieces.

7. Assemble tacos by placing pieces of mahi mahi onto warmed corn tortillas. Top with salsa and serve.

Sweet Chili Shrimp

Cooking Time: 11 minutes   Servings: 4

INGREDIENTS
√ 1 pound jumbo shrimp, peeled and deveined
√ ¼ cup sweet chili sauce
√ 1 lime, zested and juiced
√ 1 tablespoon soy sauce
√ 1 tablespoon honey
√ 1 tablespoon olive oil
√ 1 large garlic clove, minced
√ ½ teaspoon salt
√ ¼ teaspoon pepper
√ 1 green onion, thinly sliced, for garnish

DIRECTIONS

1. Place the shrimp in a large bowl. Whisk all the remaining ingredients except the green onion in a separate bowl.

2. Pour sauce over the shrimp and toss to coat.

3. Select the Preheat function on the Cosori Smart Air Fryer Toaster Oven, adjust temperature to 430°F, and press Start/Pause.

4. Line the food tray with foil, place shrimp on the tray, then insert at top position in the preheated oven.

5. Select the Air Fry function, adjust time to 6 minutes, and press Start/Pause.

6. Remove shrimp and garnish with sliced green onions.

Cinnamon Apple Chips

Cooking Time: 485 minutes   Servings: 4

INGREDIENTS

√ 1 apple
√ 1 tablespoon lemon juice
√ ¼ teaspoon cinnamon

DIRECTIONS

1. Slice the apple into ⅛-inch-thick slices, preferably by using a mandoline slicer.
2. Place slices in a bowl of water mixed with the lemon juice to prevent browning. Remove after 2 minutes and dry thoroughly with paper towels.
3. Sprinkle the apple slices with cinnamon and place on the food tray.
4. Insert the food tray at mid position in the preheated oven.
5. Select the Dehydrate function on the Cosori Smart Air Fryer Toaster Oven, adjust time to 8 hours, and press Start/Pause.
6. Remove when apple chips are crispy.

Slow Cooked Carnitas

Cooking Time: 365 minutes   Servings: 6

INGREDIENTS

√ 1 pork shoulder (5 pounds), bone-in
√ 2½ teaspoons kosher salt
√ 1½ teaspoons black pepper
√ 1½ teaspoons ground cumin
√ 1 teaspoon dried oregano
√ 1 cinnamon stick
√ 1 lime, juiced
√ ¼ teaspoon ground coriander
√ 2 bay leaves
√ 6 garlic cloves
√ 1 small onion, quartered
√ 1 full orange peel (no white)
√ 2 oranges, juiced

DIRECTIONS

1. Season the pork shoulder with salt, pepper, cumin, oregano, and coriander.
2. Place the seasoned pork shoulder in a large pot along with any seasoning that did not stick to the pork.
3. Add in the bay leaves, garlic cloves, onion, cinnamon stick, and orange peel.
4. Squeeze in the juice of two oranges and one lime and cover with foil.
5. Insert the wire rack at low position in the Cosori Smart Air Fryer Toaster Oven, then place the pot on the rack.
6. Select the Slow Cook function and press Start/Pause.
7. Remove carefully when done, uncover, and remove the bone.
8. Shred the carnitas and use them in tacos, burritos, or any other way you please.

Southwestern Stuffed Bell Peppers

Cooking Time: 60 minutes   Servings: 4

INGREDIENTS

√ 4 large bell peppers, cult in half lengthwise and seeds removed

√ 1 tablespoon olive oil

√ 1 large shallot (or 1 small onion), diced

√ 2 garlic cloves, minced

√ 1 jalapeno, seeded and finely diced

√ 1 pound ground turkey (or ground beef)

√ 1 (15 ounce) can of black beans, drained

√ 1 cup frozen corn, thawed

√ 1 ½ cups Mexican-blend cheese, shredded

√ 2 teaspoons cumin

√ 2 teaspoons chili powder

√ ½ teaspoon paprika

√ ½ teaspoon garlic powder

√ ½ teaspoon dried oregano

√ Salt and pepper to taste

√ 28 ounces diced tomatoes (in tomato juice)

√ 1 cup cooked brown rice (or white rice)

√ ¼ cup cilantro, chopped

DIRECTIONS

1. Heat a large pan over medium high heat with olive oil. Add shallot, garlic, and jalapeno. Sautee for 5 minutes or until soft. Pour mixture into a bowl.

2. Add ground turkey in the same pan. Saute until turkey is browned and cooked thoroughly.

3. Add shallot mixture back into the pan.

4. Add black beans, corn, spices, diced tomatoes, and salt and pepper to taste. Cook to reduce the tomatoes a bit and to meld the flavors. Remove from the stove and add in rice and cilantro.

5. Spoon turkey mixture into each bell pepper half.

6. Sprinkle the top with grated cheese.

7. Set the temperature on the Cosori Air Fryer to 300°F and press Start/Stop to preheat.

8. Line the fryer basket with aluminum foil.

9. Place stuffed peppers into the preheated air fryer.

10. Cook at 300°F for 30 minutes. If bell peppers are browning too fast on top cover with foil.

11. Remove with bell peppers are tender and cheese is golden and melted.

Cajun-Blackened Catfish

Cooking Time: 10 minutes   Servings: 2

INGREDIENTS
√ 2¼ teaspoons paprika
√ 1 teaspoon garlic powder
√ 1 teaspoon onion powder
√ 1 teaspoon ground dried thyme
√ 1 teaspoon ground black pepper
√ ¼ teaspoon cayenne pepper
√ ¼ teaspoon dried basil
√ ¼ teaspoon dried oregano
√ 2 catfish fillets (6 ounces)
√ Cooking Spray

DIRECTIONS
1. SELECT Preheat on the Cosori Air Fryer, adjust to 320°F, and press Start/Pause.
2. MIX all of the seasonings together in a bowl.
3. COAT the fish liberally on each side with the seasoning mix.
4. SPRAY each side of the fish with cooking spray and place into the preheated air fryer.
5. SELECT Seafood and press Start/Pause.
6. REMOVE carefully when done cooking and serve over grits.

Crispy Pork Belly

Cooking Time: 140 minutes   Servings: 6

INGREDIENTS
√ 5 liters water
√ 1 cup soy sauce
√ 2 teaspoons salt, plus more for sprinkling
√ 2 teaspoons black peppercorns
√ 1 whole garlic bulb, halved
√ 2 inch piece ginger, sliced
√ 3 green onions, cut into thirds
√ 1½ pounds pork belly

DIRECTIONS
1. Add water, soy sauce, salt, black peppercorns, garlic bulb, ginger, and green onions into a large pot and bring to a boil.
2. Place the pork belly into the seasoned broth and boil for 40 minutes uncovered. Make sure that the pork belly is fully submerged in the broth, if not add water until it is.
3. Remove the pork belly from the water and pat dry.
4. Allow the pork belly to cool for 1 hour.
5. Pierce the skin of the pork belly with a fork repeatedly all over and sprinkle with salt.
6. Select the Preheat function on the Cosori Air Fryer and press Start/Pause.
7. Place the pork belly into the preheated air fryer basket.
8. Select the Steak function, adjust time to 40 minutes, and press Start/Pause.
9. Remove the pork belly and allow to cool for 5 minutes
10. Cut and serve.

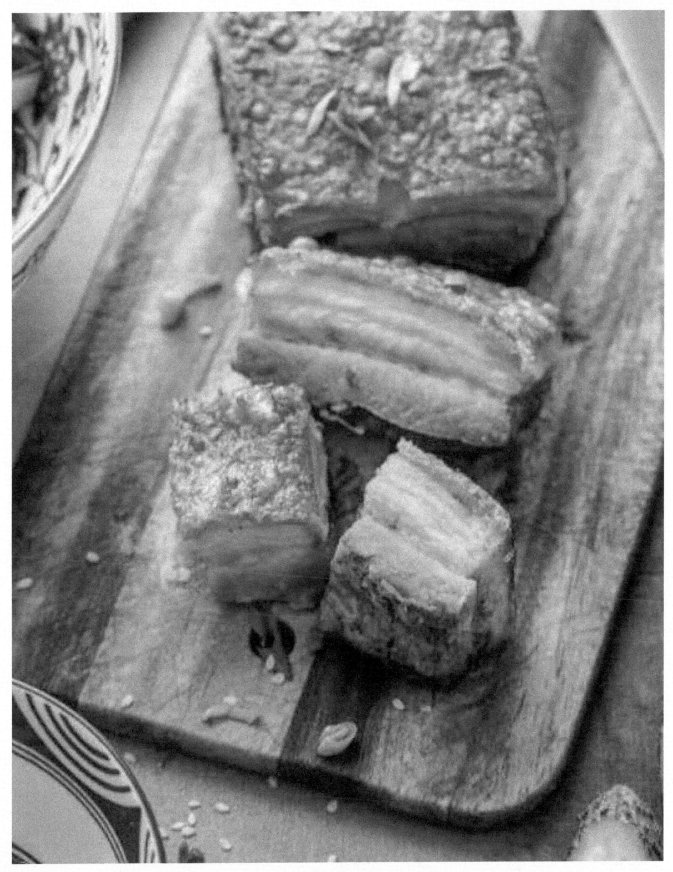

Prosciutto-Wrapped Pork Roulade

Cooking Time: 19 minutes   Servings: 4-5

INGREDIENTS
√ 6 pieces prosciutto, thinly sliced
√ 1 pork tenderloin (1 pound), halved, butterflied & pounded flat
√ 1 teaspoon salt
√ ½ teaspoon black pepper
√ 8 ounces fresh spinach leaves, divided
√ 4 slices mozzarella cheese, divided
√ 1/3 cup sun-dried tomatoes, divided
√ 2 teaspoons olive oil, divided

DIRECTIONS
1. LAY OUT 3 pieces of prosciutto on parchment, slightly overlapping one another. Place 1 pork half on the prosciutto. Repeat with the other half.
2. SEASON the inside of the pork roulades with salt and pepper.
3. LAYER half the amounts of spinach, cheese, and sun-dried tomatoes atop the pork tenderloin, leaving a ½-inch border on all sides.
4. ROLL the tenderloin around the filling tightly and tie together with kitchen string to keep closed.
5. REPEAT the process for the other pork tenderloin. Place the roulades in the fridge.
6. SELECT Preheat on the Cosori Air Fryer and press Start/Pause.
7. BRUSH 1 teaspoon of olive oil onto each wrapped tenderloin and place into the preheated air fryer.
8. SELECT Steak, adjust time to 9 minutes, and press Start/Pause.
9. ALLOW roulades to rest for 10 minutes before slicing.

Shrimp and Veggie Kebabs

Cooking Time: 23 minutes   Servings: 4

INGREDIENTS
√ ½ pound large raw shrimp, peeled and deveined
√ ½ red bell pepper
√ ½ red onion
√ 4 tablespoons olive oil
√ 2 tablespoons parsley, finely chopped
√ 4 cloves garlic, minced
√ ½ lemon, juiced
√ Salt & pepper, to taste
√ Olive oil spray
√ 6 Wooden Skewers, soaked in water for 15 minutes

DIRECTIONS
1. Soak the wooden skewers in water for 15 minutes.
2. Cut the bell peppers and red onion into 1-inch pieces.
3. Cut the wooden skewers so they fit into the air fryer. Alternately skewer the shrimp, red onion, and bell peppers until all the shrimp is used up. Spray the skewers lightly with olive oil and season with salt and pepper.
4. Select the Preheat function on the Cosori Air Fryer and press Start/Pause.
5. Place shrimp kebabs into the preheated air fryer.
6. Set temperature to 400°F and time to 8 minutes, then press Start/Pause. Flip kebabs halfway through cooking.
7. Combine the olive oil, parsley, garlic, and lemon juice in a bowl.
8. Remove the kebabs when done, brush with the lemon garlic herb mixture, and serve.

Ribs with Sweet and Spicy Mango BBQ Sauce

Cooking Time: 115 minutes   Servings: 5

INGREDIENTS

Ribs
√ 1 rack of baby back ribs
√ 2 teaspoons salt
√ 1½ teaspoons black pepper
√ 1½ teaspoons garlic powder
√ 1½ teaspoons smoked paprika

BBQ Sauce
√ 1 tablespoon olive oil
√ 1 small onion, chopped
√ 3 garlic cloves, minced
√ 1 teaspoon ginger, grated
√ 1 mango, peeled, pitted, and chopped
√ 1 cup tomato puree
√ 3 tablespoons tomato paste
√ ½ serrano chile, whole
√ 1/3 cup apple cider vinegar
√ ½ cup brown sugar
√ 2 tablespoons molasses
√ 1 tablespoon worcestershire
√ 1 tablespoon dijon mustard

DIRECTIONS

1. Remove the membrane from the ribs. Cut into sections of 4 ribs each. Dry ribs with paper towels. Season with salt, pepper, garlic powder, and smoked paprika. Wrap each section of ribs tightly in foil.

2. Insert ribs into the air fryer baskets. Set temperature to 350°F and time to 1 hour, then press Start/Pause.

3. Make the barbecue sauce by heating a pot over medium heat. Add the olive oil and onion and saute for 5 minutes. Add the garlic and ginger and saute for 30 seconds.

4. Add the mango, tomato puree, tomato paste, whole serrano chile, apple cider vinegar, brown sugar, molasses, worcestershire, dijon mustard, hot sauce, salt, pepper, and chile powder.

5. Bring to a very low boil, then reduce heat to low and simmer for 20 minutes, stirring occasionally. Remove the serrano chile and discard. Let the sauce cool slightly.

6. Puree sauce in a high speed blender until smooth. Pour sauce into a jar to store while ribs cook.

7. Remove ribs from the air fryer baskets after 1 hour and remove the foil. Brush the ribs with BBQ sauce. Place ribs back into the air fryer.

8. Set temperature to 320°F and time to 25 minutes, then press Start/Pause.

9. Flip ribs halfway through cooking and brush with additional BBQ sauce.

10. Remove when ribs are tender and caramelized.

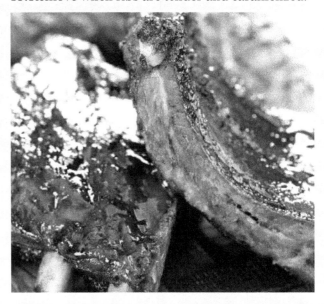

Cheesy Baked Gnocchi

Cooking Time: 25 minutes   Servings: 2

INGREDIENTS

√ 1¼ cups your favorite marinara sauce

√ 1 tablespoon olive oil

√ ½ of a (17.5 oz) package gnocchi

√ ¼ cup grated parmesan cheese

√ ¼ cup shredded mozzarella

√ 2 tablespoons fresh basil, chopped

DIRECTIONS

1. Grease a 6-inch baking dish with olive oil. Combine gnocchi, marinara sauce, basil, and parmesan cheese together in a bowl, making sure the gnocchi is evenly coated in the sauce.

2. Add gnocchi to the baking dish and sprinkle with shredded mozzarella on top.

3. Select the Preheat function on the Cosori Air Fryer, adjust temperature to 350°F, and press Start/Pause.

4. Insert the baking dish into the preheated air fryer. Set time to 10 minutes and press Start/Pause.

5. Lower temperature to 300°F and bake for 5 more minutes.

6. Remove when cheese is browned and sauce is bubbly.

7. Allow gnocchi to rest for 10 minutes before serving.

North Carolina Style Pork Chops

Cooking Time: 15 minutes   Servings: 2

INGREDIENTS

√ 2 pork chops, boneless

√ 2 teaspoons vegetable oil

√ 2 tablespoons dark brown sugar, packed

√ 2 teaspoons Hungarian paprika

√ 1 teaspoon ground mustard

√ 1 teaspoon freshly ground black pepper

√ 1 teaspoon onion powder

√ 1 teaspoon garlic powder

√ Salt & pepper, to taste

DIRECTIONS

1. SELECT Preheat on the Cosori Air Fryer and press Start/Pause.

2. COAT the pork chops with oil.

3. COMBINE all the spices and liberally season the pork chops, almost as if it were breading.

4. PLACE the pork chops into the preheated air fryer.

5. SELECT Steak, adjust to 10 minutes, and press Start/Pause.

6. REMOVE the pork chops when done cooking, allow to rest for 5 minutes, then serve.

Filipino Adobo Chicken Wings

INGREDIENTS

√ 1½ cups low-sodium soy sauce
√ ½ cup white distilled vinegar
√ 1 tablespoon mirin
√ ½ brown onion, sliced
√ 12 garlic cloves, smashed
√ 2 bay leaves
√ 2 pounds chicken wings
√ 1 tablespoon vegetable oil
√ 3 tablespoons water
√ Freshly chopped green onions, for garnish
√ Steam jasmine rice, for serving

DIRECTIONS

1. Mix together the soy sauce, vinegar, mirin, sliced onion, garlic, black pepper, and bay leaves in a resealable plastic bag.
2. Add the chicken wings and marinate in the fridge for 8 hours or overnight.
3. Remove the chicken wings from the marinade and set aside.
4. Select the Preheat function, adjust to 360°F, and press Start/Pause.
5. Place the chicken wings in the preheated air fryer basket.
6. Adjust the temperature to 360°F, set time to 22 minutes, and press Start/Pause. Flip the wings halfway through cooking.
7. Pour the marinade into a saucepan and cook on medium heat until it reaches a simmer, about 5 minutes.

8. Pour in the vegetable oil and water into the saucepan and mix well. and simmer for 15 minutes.
9. Remove the wings when done cooking and pour off any of the rendered fat into the sauce. Mix well.
10. Garnish the chicken wings with green onions.
11. Serve steam rice and the sauce on the side. (It is customary to mix sauce with rice.)

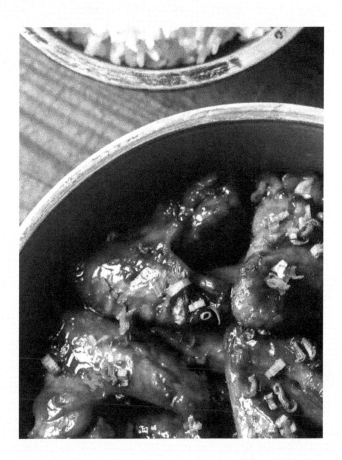

Beer and Bacon Mac and Cheese

Cooking Time: 43 minutes   Servings: 4

INGREDIENTS

√ 4 slices thick-cut bacon
√ 8 ounces uncooked macaroni
√ ½ cup beer (imperial stout)
√ 2 cups chicken stock
√ 2 teaspoons dijon mustard
√ 1 teaspoon worcestershire sauce
√ ¼ teaspoon freshly ground black pepper
√ ½ teaspoon garlic powder
√ 1 teaspoon onion powder
√ ¼ teaspoon cayenne pepper
√ A pinch ground white pepper
√ A pinch ground clove
√ A pinch ground nutmeg
√ ½ cup warm heavy cream
√ 1¾ cup shredded sharp cheddar cheese, divided
√ ¾ cup shredded low-moisture part skim mozzarella cheese, divided

DIRECTIONS

1. Select the Preheat function on the Cosori Air Fryer, adjust to 320F, and press Start/Pause.
2. Place the bacon slices in the preheated air fryer basket.
3. Select the Bacon function and press Start/Pause.
4. Remove the bacon when done and cut into bits.
5. Mix together bacon bits, ½ cup sharp cheddar cheese, and ¼ cup mozzarella cheese until well combined. Set aside.
6. Pour the bacon fat into the cake pan accessory.
7. Mix together uncooked macaroni, beer, chicken stock, mustard, worcestershire sauce, salt, blac pepper, garlic powder, onion powder, cayenne pepper, white pepper, ground clove, and clove nutmeg in the cake pan accessory until well combined.
8. Select the Preheat function on the Cosori Air Fryer, adjust to 360°F, and press Start/Pause.
9. Place the cake pan accessory in the preheated air fryer basket.
10. Adjust the temperature to 360°F, set time for 22 minutes, and press Start/Pause. Stir the macaroni two times during cooking.
11. Add warm heavy cream, 1½ cup sharp cheddar cheese, and ½ cup mozzarella cheese into the cooked macaroni until the cheese is melted.
12. Top the macaroni and cheese with the bacon and cheese mixture, and place back into the air fryer.
13. Adjust the temperature to 360°F, set time for 3 minutes, and press Start/Pause.

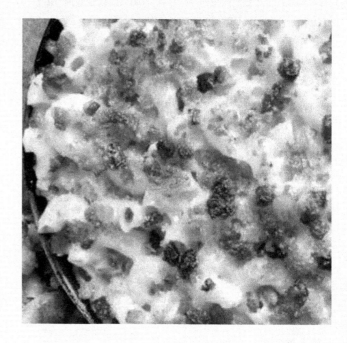

APPETIZER RECIPES

Peanut Butter Pizookie

INGREDIENTS

√ 255 grams (2 cups plus 2 tablespoons) all-purpose flour

√ 7 grams (1¼ teaspoon) baking soda

√ 3 grams of (½ teaspoon) kosher salt

√ 225 grams (1 cup) unsalted butter, softened, plus more for greasing

√ 225 grams (2 cups) light brown sugar

√ 225 grams (2 cups white granulated sugar)

√ 115 grams eggs (about 3 extra-large eggs), whisked

√ 3 grams (½ teaspoon) vanilla

√ 340 grams (1½ cups) peanut butter (chunky or smooth)

√ 145 grams (1½ cups) roasted peanuts, optional

√ Items Needed:

√ Stand mixer fitted with paddle attachment

√ Cosori Pizza Pan accessory

√ Cake tester or toothpick

√ Wire rack

DIRECTIONS

1. Sift the flour, baking soda, and salt into a large bowl and stir to combine.

2. Cream the butter and sugars together on medium speed in the bowl of a stand mixer fitted with the paddle attachment until smooth, pale, and fluffy, about 5 minutes.

3. Combine the whisked eggs with the vanilla, then add to the creamed butter in 3 additions while mixing on medium speed until fully incorporated.

4. Add the peanut butter while mixing on medium speed until fully incorporated.

5. Add the sifted dry ingredients while mixing on low speed until just combined.

6. Divide the cookie dough into 4 equal pieces.

7. Grease the pizza pan accessory with butter and sprinkle with flour, then flip over and tap out excess flour.

8. Roll the dough pieces into balls and place them into the pizza pan accessory. Press down on each ball to flatten slightly.

9. Select the Preheat function on the Cosori Air Fryer, adjust temperature to 320°F, then press Start/Pause.

10. Place the pizza pan accessory into the preheated air fryer.

11. Set temperature to 320°F and time to 15 minutes, then press Start/Pause.

12. Insert a cake tester or toothpick into the center of the pizookies when the timer goes off. If it comes out clean, it is done. If there is still dough sticking to the tester, cook for an additional 2 minutes.

13. Cool the pizookie while still in the pizza pan accessory on a wire rack for 5 minutes.

14. Remove the pizookie from the pizza pan accessory, transfer to a plate, and top with ice cream and other desired toppings.

15. Serve immediately.

Chocolate Chunk Pizookie

INGREDIENTS

√ 300 grams (2½ cups scant) all-purpose flour

√ 7 grams (1¼ teaspoon) baking soda

√ 5 grams (1 teaspoon) kosher salt

√ 200 grams (½ cup plus 2 tablespoons) unsalted butter, softened, plus more for greasing

√ 140 grams (2/3 cup) white granulated sugar

√ 90 grams (1/3 cup) light brown sugar

√ 85 grams eggs (about 2 eggs), whisked

√ 3 grams (½ teaspoon) vanilla

√ 300 grams (2 cups) chocolate chunks or large chocolate chips

√ Ice cream of your choice, for topping (optional)

Items Needed:

√ Stand mixer fitted with paddle attachment

√ Cosori Pizza Pan accessory

√ Cake tester or toothpick

√ Wire rack

DIRECTIONS

1. Sift the flour, baking soda, and salt, into a large bowl and stir to combine. Set aside.

2. Cream the butter and sugars together on medium speed in the bowl of a stand mixer fitted with the paddle attachment until smooth, pale, and fluffy, about 5 minutes.

3. Combine the whisked eggs with the vanilla, then add to the creamed butter in 3 additions while mixing on medium speed until fully incorporated.

4. Add the sifted dry ingredients and chocolate chunks while mixing on low speed until just incorporated.

5. Divide the cookie dough into 3 equal pieces.

6. Grease the pizza pan accessory with butter and sprinkle with flour, then flip over and tap out excess flour.

7. Roll the dough into balls and place them into the pizza pan accessory. Press down on each ball to flatten slightly.

8. Select the Preheat function on the Cosori Air Fryer, adjust temperature to 330°F, then press Start/Pause.

9. Place the pizza pan accessory into the preheated air fryer.

10. Set temperature to 330°F and time to 14 minutes, then press Start/Pause.

11. Insert a cake tester or toothpick into the center of the pizookie when the timer goes off. If it comes out clean, it is done. If there is still dough sticking to the tester, cook for an additional 2 minutes.

12. Remove when done and cool the pizookie while still in the pizza pan accessory on a wire rack for 5 minutes.

13. Remove the pizookie from the pizza pan accessory, transfer to a plate, and top with ice cream and other desired toppings.

14. Serve immediately.

Guinness® Crème Brûlée

INGREDIENTS

√ 2 cups heavy cream
√ 2 cups Guinness® beer
√ 1 cup granulated sugar, divided
√ 1 tablespoon vanilla extract
√ 6 large egg yolks
√ 1 cup hot water
√ Berries, for garnish
√ Mint, for garnish
√ Items Needed:
√ Electric hand mixer
√ 4 ramekins (10 ounces)
√ Square aluminum foil pan (6 x 6 inches)
√ Butane kitchen torch

DIRECTIONS

1. Combine the heavy cream, Guinness® beer, and 1/3 cup of sugar into a medium saucepan over medium-high heat and bring to a boil. Reduce heat and simmer for 5 minutes.
2. Cream the vanilla extract, 1/3 cup sugar, and egg yolks together using an electric hand mixer until light and fluffy.
3. Pour the Guinness® mixture slowly into the egg mixture while whisking at low speed. Whisk until fully incorporated and smooth.
4. Divide the mixture into 4 ramekins.
5. Cut the ridged rim off the aluminum foil pan and set aside.
6. Select the Preheat function on the Cosori Air Fryer, adjust temperature to 300°F, then press Start/Pause.
7. Insert the aluminum foil pan into the preheated air fryer.

8. Add 1 cup of hot water to the bottom of the aluminum foil pan, then place 2 ramekins into the pan.
9. Set temperature to 300°F and time to 40 minutes, then press Start/Pause.
10. Remove the crème brûlée when the custard is set. It should jiggle but not be liquid.
11. Cool the crème brûlée completely in the refrigerator, about 2 hours.
12. Remove the crème brûlée from the refrigerator and let come to room temperature, about 30 minutes.
13. Divide the remaining 1/3 cup of sugar amongst the 4 ramekins and spread evenly on top. Gently tap out the excess sugar. Carefully use a kitchen torch to melt the sugar and form a crispy top.
14. Allow the crème brûlée to cool and set for 5 minutes before serving.
15. Garnish the tops of the crème brûlée with berries and mint and serve immediately.

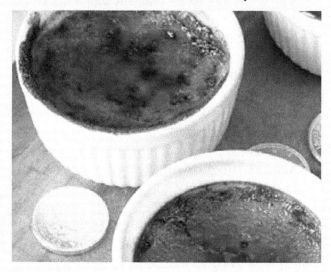

Meatball Sliders

INGREDIENTS

Sliders:
√ 3 tablespoons unsalted butter
√ 4 cloves garlic, minced
√ 9 store-bought pull-apart dinner rolls
√ 1 cup prepared tomato sauce
√ ½ cup shredded Italian cheese blend
√ 2 tablespoons fresh basil, chopped

Meatballs:
√ 2 tablespoons olive oil
√ 1 small onion, finely diced
√ 3 cloves garlic, minced
√ ½ teaspoon red pepper flakes
√ 1 pound grass-fed ground beef
√ 2 tablespoons fresh parsley, finely chopped
√ 1 large egg
√ ¼ cup plain breadcrumbs
√ 1/4 cup Parmesan cheese, freshly grated
√ 1½ teaspoons kosher salt
√ 1 teaspoon black pepper
√ Olive oil spray

DIRECTIONS

1. Place olive oil in a small skillet over medium heat to start the meatballs.

2. Add the diced onion and sauté until translucent and lightly golden, about 3 minutes.

3. Add the minced garlic and red pepper flakes and sauté for another minute.

4. Remove the skillet from the heat and let cool to room temperature.

5. Transfer the cooled onions and garlic to a large bowl.

6. Add the beef, parsley, egg, breadcrumbs, Parmesan cheese, salt, and pepper, and mix with your hands until well combined.

7. Shape all of the mixture into 2-inch balls.

8. Select the Preheat function on the Cosori Smart Air Fryer, then press Start/Pause.

9. Place the meatballs into the preheated air fryer and lightly spray the tops with oil spray.

10. Set temperature to 400°F and time to 12 minutes, then press Start/Pause.

11. Remove the meatballs when done and transfer to a plate.

Note: Clean the air fryer basket before continuing.

12. Place butter in a small skillet over medium heat to start the sliders.

13. Add the minced garlic once the butter is sizzling, then turn off the heat. Let the garlic infuse the butter for 5 minutes.

14. Cut a 2-inch-diameter circle into the top of each roll without cutting all the way through, creating a well. Discard the removed bread.

15. Brush the garlic butter over the outside and inside of each roll.

16. Line the air fryer basket with foil that goes up the sides of the basket.

17. Place the rolls into the air fryer basket.

18. Set temperature to 400°F and time to 5 minutes, then press Start/Pause.

19. Remove the rolls when golden brown and lightly toasted.

20. Place 1 tablespoon of tomato sauce into the bottom of each well, then place the meatballs on top.

21. Top each meatball with another tablespoon of tomato sauce and sprinkle cheese over the whole roll.

22. Set temperature to 400°F and time to 2 minutes, then press Start/Pause.

23. Remove the sliders when done and the cheese is melted and golden.

24. Serve the sliders warm, topped with fresh basil.

INGREDIENTS

Dumpling Filling:
√ 1 head Napa cabbage
√ 1 tablespoon plus 2 teaspoons kosher salt
√ 1 pound ground pork
√ 1 pound shrimp, sized 41/50, peeled, head removed, and deveined
√ 1 bunch Chinese chives, finely chopped
√ 1 bunch green onions, finely chopped
√ ½-inch piece fresh ginger, peeled and minced
√ 2 tablespoons soy sauce
√ 1½ teaspoons sesame oil
√ ¼ teaspoon white pepper

Dumpling Wrapping:
√ All-purpose flour, as needed
√ 1 cup water, plus more as needed
√ 2 packages dumpling wrappers, room temperature
√ Oil spray, to turn into potstickers

For Serving:
√ Soy sauce
√ Sambal
√ Black vinegar
√ ¼-inch piece fresh ginger, peeled & julienned
√ Items Needed:
√ 3 half-sheet baking pans

DIRECTIONS

1. Wash the cabbage by gently pulling apart the leaves and rinsing each layer.
2. Arrange the cabbage leaves horizontally onto a cutting board and cut into 2-inch-long, ¼-inch-thick pieces. Place into a large bowl.
3. Sprinkle 1 tablespoon of kosher salt over the cabbage, mix well, and let sit for 10 minutes.
4. Squeeze the cabbage over a large colander to wring out excess moisture and catch any pieces that fall out. Set aside.
5. Add the pork, shrimp, Chinese chives, green onions, cabbage, and ginger to a large mixing bowl and mix well.

6. Add soy sauce, sesame oil, white pepper, and 2 teaspoons salt to the mixing bowl, and mix well.
7. Lay plastic wrap onto a clean surface for your wrapping station and sprinkle a small amount of flour across the entire surface. Prepare 3 half-sheet baking pans by sprinkling flour onto each and setting aside.
8. Set up your wrapping station by arranging the dumpling filling, 1 cup of water, and the room temperature dumpling wrappers in the middle of your working surface.
9. Place one wrapper completely flat in the palm of your hand. Place a minimum of 2 teaspoons of filling in the center of the wrapper.
10. Dip your pinky or index finger into the water and circle the edge of the wrapper.
11. Fold the wrapper in half and pinch the sides in, forming a half moon with triangles on each end to seal.
Note: For a visual guide on sealing dumplings, see our Cooking with Cosori video.
12. Place the completed dumplings onto the floured baking sheets, continuing with the remaining filling and wrappers.

To Cook as Dumplings:
13. Fill a large pot halfway with water and bring to a boil.
14. Add 15 dumplings at a time to the water. Allow the water to come back to a boil, then lower heat to a medium simmer.
15. Cook the dumplings until done, about 8 minutes.
16. Remove the dumplings from the water when done and place on a clean plate.
17. Serve immediately with a side of soy sauce and sambal to enjoy as dumplings.

To Cook as Potstickers:
18. Select the Preheat function on the Cosori Air Fryer, set temperature to 380°F, and press Start/Pause.
19. Spray the preheated inner air fryer basket and

dumplings with oil spray.

20. Place 12 dumplings (frozen or cooked) into the inner air fryer basket. You will need to work in batches.

21. Set temperature to 380°F and time to 10 minutes, press Shake, then press Start/Pause.

22. Flip the potstickers over and spray with oil spray halfway through cooking. The Shake Reminder will let you know when.

23. Remove the potstickers from the air fryer when done.

24. Repeat the cooking process with the remaining dumplings.

25. Serve immediately with a side of soy sauce, sambal, black vinegar, and fresh ginger.

Note: Freeze the remaining dumplings or potstickers on baking sheets overnight, then transfer into an airtight bag or container to store. The frozen dumplings or potstickers have a shelf life of 1 month and are best eaten within 3 weeks of freezing.

Rustic Mediterranean Tomato Dip with Grilled Pita

Cooking Time: 11 minutes   Servings: 4

INGREDIENTS
√ 4 pitas
√ 8 ounces grape tomatoes
√ 1/3 cup kalamata olives, pitted and chopped
√ 2 tablespoons pine nuts
√ 2 tablespoons fresh mint leaves, chopped
√ ½ tablespoon fresh dill, chopped
√ 1 teaspoon dried oregano
√ 1 garlic clove, very finely minced
√ 1 tablespoon red wine vinegar
√ 2 tablespoons olive oil, divided
√ ½ teaspoon freshly ground black pepper
√ Kosher salt, to taste
√ 16 ounces labneh

DIRECTIONS
1. Place the cooking pot into the base of the Cosori Indoor Grill, followed by the grill grate.

2. Select the Air Grill function on low heat, adjust time to 5 minutes, press Shake, then press Start/Pause to preheat.

3. Place the pitas onto the preheated grill grate, then close the lid.

4. Flip the pitas over halfway through the cooking time. The Shake Reminder will let you know when.

5. Remove the pitas and set aside.

6. Place the tomatoes onto the grill grate, then close the lid.

7. Select the Air Grill function on medium heat, adjust time to 6 minutes, press the Preheat button to bypass the preheat function, then press Start/Pause to begin cooking.

8. Transfer the grilled tomatoes to a bowl with the olives, pine nuts, chopped herbs, oregano, garlic, vinegar, 1 tablespoon olive oil, and black pepper. Stir together until combined, then season to taste with kosher salt.

9. Scoop the labneh into a serving bowl, top with the tomato mixture, drizzle with the remaining olive oil, and serve with the pita bread for dipping.

Arancini

INGREDIENTS

√ 5 cups low-sodium chicken stock
√ 4 tablespoons unsalted butter, divided
√ 1 medium onion, finely chopped
√ 1½ teaspoons kosher salt, plus more for seasoning
√ 3 garlic cloves, minced
√ 1 cup Arborio rice
√ ½ cup dry white wine
√ ¾ cup Parmigiano Reggiano, freshly grated
√ 2 teaspoons lemon zest
√ ¼ cup frozen peas
√ 1 teaspoon black pepper, plus more for seasoning
√ 2 ounces low-moisture mozzarella, cut into 1/3-inch pieces
√ 2 cups panko breadcrumbs
√ ½ cup all-purpose flour
√ 2 eggs
√ Olive oil spray

Items Needed:
√ Food Processor

DIRECTIONS

1. Place the chicken stock in a medium pot and bring to a simmer over medium heat. Once simmering, keep warm over low heat.

2. Place 2 tablespoons of butter in a medium saucepan over medium heat.

3. Add the onion and salt and cook until softened, about 4 minutes. Add the garlic and cook for 1 more minute.

4. Add the rice and stir until the rice is fully coated in the butter and starts to turn translucent around the edges, about 3 minutes.

5. Add the wine and cook, stirring often, until the pan is almost dry. Ladle in 1 cup of the warm chicken stock until the rice is just covered.

6. Cook stirring often, until the chicken stock is just above the surface of the rice, keeping the liquid at a consistent low boil. Repeat this process until you have added all of the chicken stock and the risotto is cooked through.

7. Remove the risotto from the heat and add the Parmigiano Reggiano, lemon zest, remaining butter, peas, pepper, and salt to taste.

8. Spread the risotto in an even layer on a baking sheet lined with parchment paper. Chill in the refrigerator for 1 to 2 hours.

9. Scoop the risotto into ¼ cup portions and form into 2-inch balls.

10. Stuff 2 to 3 pieces of mozzarella into the center of each ball, sealing any holes. Place the risotto balls onto a baking sheet lined with parchment paper and freeze for 10 minutes.

11. Place the panko breadcrumbs into a food processor and pulse until the crumbs become fine. Transfer the breadcrumbs to a shallow dish.

12. Place the flour in a separate shallow dish and season lightly with salt and pepper. Beat the eggs in a third separate shallow dish.

13. Select the Preheat function on the Cosori Air Fryer, adjust temperature to 380°F, and press Start/Pause.

14. Remove the risotto balls from the freezer.

15. Dredge each risotto ball in the flour, shaking off any excess. Then, evenly coat the risotto balls with the egg mixture, followed by the breadcrumbs.

16. Spray the risotto balls evenly on all sides with olive oil spray.

17. Place the arancini into the preheated air fryer basket.

18. Set temperature to 380°F and time to 15 minutes, then press Start/Pause.

19. Remove the arancini when golden brown and serve immediately.

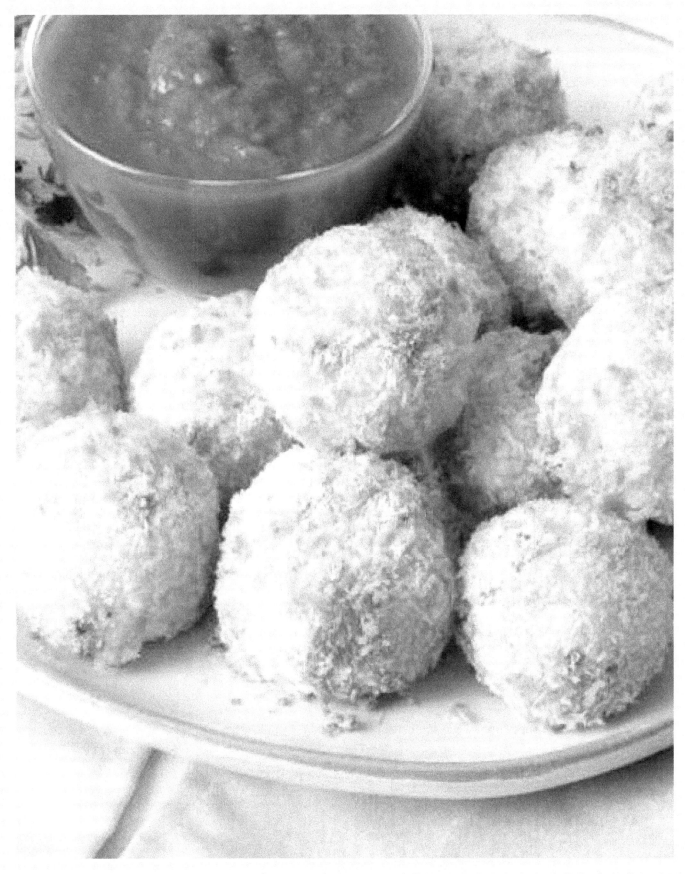

Challah Bread

INGREDIENTS

√ 1 pound bread flour
√ 6 grams instant dry yeast
√ 6 fluid ounces of water
√ 90 grams egg yolks (about 5 yolks)
√ 46 grams vegetable oil

Items Needed:
√ Stand Mixer
√ Kitchen scale
√ 46 grams white granulated sugar
√ 8 grams kosher salt
√ Egg wash (yolks only), for brushing, plus more as needed
√ Bread flour, for dusting, plus more as needed

DIRECTIONS

1. Combine the flour and yeast. Separately, add the water, egg yolks, oil, sugar, and salt into the bowl of the stand mixer. Then, add in the flour-yeast mixture.

2. Mix with the dough hook attachment on low speed for 4 minutes and then on medium speed for 4 minutes. The dough should be slightly firm and smooth, but not sticky.

3. Proof the dough until doubled, about 1 hour.

4. Divide the dough into 6 separate 130-gram pieces. Shape into oblongs and allow the dough to rest, covered, for about 10 to 15 minutes to let the gluten rest.

5. Fold the dough into thirds, then shape each third into a long rope about 24-inches long.

6. Cut each rope into 3 smaller ropes, about 8-inches long each. You should have a total of 18, 8-inch ropes.

Note: Make sure the ropes are all the same size, so your braid comes out evenly.

7. Dust the tops of the ropes lightly with bread flour.

8. Braid by pinching the tops of the ropes together and, beginning in the center of the strands, place the left strand over the center strand, then the right strand over the center strand. Repeat until you reach the end of the dough.

9. Pinch together the ends of the braids to seal.

10. Place the braided Challah on parchment lined sheet pans dusted lightly with bread flour.

11. Brush the completed braids with egg yolk wash.

12. Proof the dough, covered, until the dough springs back halfway, slowly to the touch, but does not collapse, about 1 hour.

13. Brush the dough again with the egg yolk wash before baking.

14. Select the Preheat function on the Cosori Air Fryer, adjust temperature to 300°F, and press Start/Pause.

15. Line the inner air fryer basket with parchment paper, being careful of hot surfaces.

16. Place the Challah braids into the preheated basket.

17. Set temperature to 300°F and time to 15 minutes, then press Start/Pause.

18. Remove when done and let cool completely on a wire rack.

19. Serve immediately.

Spider Pretzel Dip Bowl

INGREDIENTS

√ 2 tablespoons dark brown sugar

√ 2¼ teaspoons active dry yeast

√ 3 ounces unsalted butter, melted (90—105°F)

√ 2½ teaspoons kosher salt, plus more for topping

√ 4½ cups all-purpose flour

√ ¼ cup baking soda

√ 1 egg, beaten

√ Oil spray

√ Marinara sauce, warmed

√ 4 pimento stuffed olives, cut in half horizontally

DIRECTIONS

1. Combine 1½ cups warm water (90—105°F), dark brown sugar, butter, and yeast in a large bowl and allow to sit for 5 minutes.

2. Add the salt and flour and mix to form a dough. Knead for 10 minutes by hand or in a stand mixer with the dough hook attachment. Place dough into a lightly greased bowl, cover, and allow to rise for 1 hour.

3. Divide the dough in half then take the first halved piece and split into 8 equal pieces. Roll each piece into a long rope about 6 inches long, then set aside. Take the other halved piece and cut into two separate pieces for the head and body.

4. Fold aluminum foil into 5-inch-long rods and spray with oil spray.

5. Wrap the leg pieces around aluminum foil rods.

6. Place the 3 quarts of water and baking soda in a large pot and bring to a boil.

7. Boil pretzel pieces for 30 seconds and then place them onto a baking sheet lined with parchment paper.

8. Select the Preheat function on the Cosori Air Fryer, adjust temperature to 380°F, and press Start/Pause.

9. Brush the shaped pretzel pieces with the beaten egg and sprinkle the tops with coarse salt.

10. Place the "head" of the spider into the preheated air fryer basket.

11. Set temperature to 380°F, time to 8 minutes, enable the Shake function and press Start/Pause.

12. Flip the "head" when the Shake reminder goes off.

13. Remove from air fryer and let it cool on a wire rack off to the side and continue to bake the other parts of the spider.

14. Bake the "body" of the spider at 380F for 12 minutes, flipping halfway through the cooking process. Remove from air fryer and let cool on the wire rack.

15. Bake the "legs" of the spiders at 380F for 6 minutes, flipping halfway through the cooking process. 4 legs can fit into the air fryer basket at one time. Set on wire rack to cool.

16. Remove the foil rods carefully from the leg pieces.

17. Cut a circle into the top of the "body" of the spider and hallow out the center of the bread bowl and fill with warmed marina sauce.

18. Assemble the spider by placing the legs onto the desired plate or cutting board. Make sure there are 4 legs on each side then place the body of the spider on top of the legs. Cut a notch into the back of the "head" of the spider and place flush against the body.

Crab Cakes with Lemon Aioli

Cooking Time: 8 minutes   Servings: 6

INGREDIENTS

Crab Cakes:
√ 1 large egg
√ 1½ teaspoons Old Bay® Seasoning
√ 2 teaspoons Worcestershire sauce
√ ¼ teaspoon cayenne pepper
√ ¼ cup mayonnaise
√ 1 teaspoon Dijon mustard
√ 2 cloves garlic, minced
√ 1 teaspoon kosher salt
√ 1 pound jumbo lump crab meat, squeezed dry & picked through for shells
√ 1 cup panko breadcrumbs
√ Oil spray, as needed

Lemon Aioli:
√ ½ cup mayonnaise
√ ½ teaspoon lemon zest
√ 3 tablespoons lemon juice, fresh squeezed
√ 1 garlic clove, minced
√ ½ tablespoon chives, chopped
√ Salt & pepper, to taste

DIRECTIONS

1. Combine the egg, Old Bay® Seasoning, Worcestershire sauce, cayenne pepper, mayonnaise, Dijon mustard, garlic, and salt in a large bowl and whisk until smooth.

2. Add the crab meat and panko and gently fold the mixture together until combined, being careful not to shred the crab meat.

3. Form mixture into 6 medium-sized patties.

4. Place the mixture in the refrigerator for 30 minutes.

5. Select the Preheat function on the Cosori Air Fryer, adjust temperature to 380°F, and press Start/Pause.

6. Spray the air fryer baskets with spray oil, then arrange the crab cakes in a single layer inside the baskets. Spray the crab cakes with a light coat of spray oil.

7. Set temperature to 380°F and time to 8 minutes, then press Start/Pause.

8. Whisk together the lemon aioli ingredients in a medium bowl. Season to taste with salt and pepper and set aside.

9. Remove the crab cakes when done and serve immediately with the lemon aioli on the side.

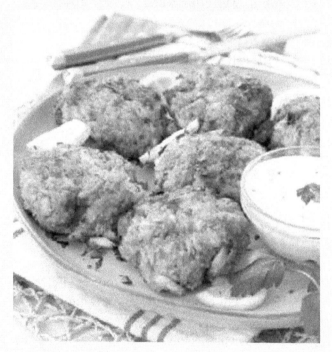

Chili Cumin Wings with Mango Cilantro Raita

Cooking Time: 20 minutes   Servings: 4

INGREDIENTS

Chili Cumin Wings:

√ 1 tablespoon grapeseed oil
√ 1 teaspoon chili powder
√ 1 tablespoon ground coriander
√ 1½ teaspoon ground cumin
√ 2 teaspoons paprika
√ ¼ teaspoon ground ginger
√ ½ teaspoon cayenne pepper
√ 2 teaspoons kosher salt
√ 2 pounds chicken wings

Mango Raita:

√ 1 cup Greek yogurt
√ ¼ cup fresh mango, small diced
√ 1 tablespoon grapeseed oil
√ 1 lime, zested & juiced
√ 2 tablespoons fresh cilantro, chopped
√ 1 tablespoon fresh mint leaves, chopped
√ Kosher salt, to taste
√ Black pepper, to taste

DIRECTIONS

1. Select the Preheat function the Cosori Air Fryer, adjust temperature to 380°F, and press Start/Pause.

2. Whisk together the grapeseed oil, chili powder, coriander, cumin, paprika, ginger, cayenne pepper, and salt in a large bowl.

3. Dry the chicken wings thoroughly with paper towels, then toss them in the bowl with the seasoning until evenly coated.

4. Arrange the wings in a single layer inside the air fryer baskets, skin side down.

5. Set temperature to 380°F and time to 20 minutes, press Shake, then press Start/Pause.

6. Flip the wings halfway through cooking. The Shake Reminder will let you know when.

7. Whisk together the raita ingredients, and then season to taste with salt and pepper.

8. Remove the wings from the air fryer when done and serve immediately with the mango raita on the side.

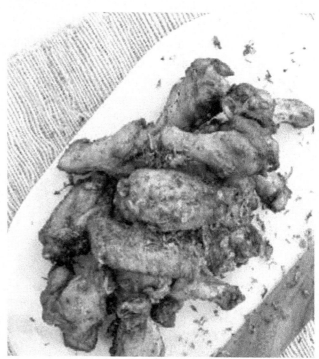

Artichoke Wings with Vegan Ranch Dip

Cooking Time: 10 minutes   Servings: 6

INGREDIENTS
Artichoke Wings
√ One 16-ounce jar marinated artichoke hearts

√ 1½ cups all-purpose flour

√ 1 teaspoon garlic powder

√ 1 teaspoon onion powder

√ 1 teaspoon paprika

√ 1 teaspoon kosher salt

√ One 12-ounce bottle beer (Lager or Weisse-style for best results)

√ 2 cups panko breadcrumbs

Vegan Ranch Dip
√ 1 cup vegan mayonnaise

√ ¼ cup non-dairy milk (i.e., coconut, oat, or any nut milk)

√ 2 tablespoons fresh dill, finely chopped

√ 1 teaspoon fresh Italian parsley leaves, finely chopped

√ 1 teaspoon vegan Worcestershire sauce (optional)

√ 1 teaspoon apple cider vinegar

√ 1 teaspoon lemon juice

√ 1 clove garlic, grated

√ 1 teaspoon onion powder

√ 1 teaspoon black pepper

√ Kosher salt, to taste

√ Oil spray

DIRECTIONS
1. Select the Preheat function on the Cosori Air Fryer then press Start/Pause.
2. Drain the artichoke hearts and pat dry with paper towels.
3. Whisk together the flour, garlic powder, onion powder, paprika, and salt in a large bowl until evenly distributed.
4. Pour in the beer and whisk well until no lumps remain. The mixture should resemble pancake batter.
5. Place the panko breadcrumbs in a separate medium bowl.
6. Line the preheated air fryer baskets with parchment paper.
7. Dredge the artichoke hearts in the beer batter, then roll in the panko breadcrumbs.
8. Shake off any excess breadcrumbs, then place the dredged artichoke hearts into the lined air fryer baskets.
9. Spray the wings lightly with oil and insert into the preheated air fryer.
10. Adjust temperature to 400°F and time to 10 minutes, press Shake, then press Start/Pause.
11. Flip the wings and spray again halfway through cooking. The Shake Reminder will let you know when.
12. Combine all the dressing ingredients in a separate medium bowl and whisk together.
13. Season to taste with kosher salt. Pour into a bowl for dipping.
14. Remove the artichoke wings from the air fryer when done.
15. Serve immediately with the vegan ranch dressing.

Buffalo Chicken Dip Bites

Cooking Time: 10 minutes   Servings: 20

INGREDIENTS

Buffalo Chicken Bites
√ 1 fully cooked rotisserie chicken
√ 4 ounces cream cheese, softened
√ 1½ cups cheddar cheese, shredded
√ 1/3 cup hot sauce (e.g., Frank's Red Hot)
√ 2 tablespoons buttermilk
√ 2 teaspoons dried dill
√ 2 teaspoons dried parsley
√ 1 teaspoon onion powder
√ 1 teaspoon garlic powder
√ 1 teaspoon cayenne pepper
√ 1 teaspoon black pepper
√ 1 teaspoon kosher salt
√ ½ cup all-purpose flour
√ 3 large eggs, beaten
√ 1½ cups panko breadcrumbs
√ Oil spray
√ 2 tablespoons chopped green onion, for garnish
√ Cut vegetables, for serving (optional)

Bleu Cheese Dip
√ 1 cup bleu cheese crumbles
√ ½ cup sour cream
√ 1/3 cup mayonnaise
√ ¼ cup buttermilk
√ 2 tablespoons chives, chopped
√ 1 tablespoon lemon juice
√ Salt & pepper, to taste

DIRECTIONS

1. Select the Preheat function on the Cosori Air Fryer, set temperature to 380°F, then press Start/Pause.

2. Remove all the meat from the rotisserie chicken, shred it, then place in a large bowl.

3. Add the cream cheese, cheddar cheese, hot sauce, buttermilk, dill, parsley, onion powder, garlic powder, cayenne, black pepper and salt to the chicken, then stir to combine thoroughly.

4. Form the chicken mixture into balls 2-inches in diameter.

5. Set up a breading station in the following order: flour, eggs, breadcrumbs. Dip each ball first into the flour, then the eggs, then the breadcrumbs, shaking off excess each time.

6. Place the breaded balls onto a parchment lined baking sheet, continuing to form the balls until all the chicken mixture has been used up.

7. Spray each ball with cooking spray lightly on all sides, then arrange 9-12 balls in the preheated air fryer baskets. Place any remaining balls into the refrigerator to reserve for a second batch.

8. Set temperature to 380°F and time to 10 minutes, then press Start/Pause.

9. Stir together the bleu cheese dip ingredients in a medium bowl, then season to taste with salt and pepper. Set aside.

10. Remove the buffalo chicken bites from the air fryer when done. Sprinkle with green onions for garnish and serve immediately with the bleu cheese dip and cut vegetables.

Chicken Satay with Peanut Sauce

Cooking Time: 27 minutes   Servings: 8

INGREDIENTS

Marinade
√ 1/3 cup coconut milk
√ 1 stalk lemongrass, chopped
√ 2 cloves garlic, peeled and smashed
√ 2 tbsp fish sauce
√ 1 tbsp fresh ginger, grated
√ 1 tbsp agave syrup or granulated sugar
√ 1 shallot, sliced
√ 1 tsp ground coriander
√ 1 tsp turmeric
√ 1 tsp chili powder
√ 1 tsp kosher salt
√ 2 lb boneless skinless chicken thighs, cut into 1" pieces

Peanut Sauce
√ ¼ cup creamy peanut butter
√ 2 tbsp soy sauce or tamari
√ 2 tbsp fresh lime juice
√ 1 tbsp grated fresh ginger
√ 2 tsp agave syrup or granulated sugar
√ 1 tsp kosher salt
√ Water, as needed
√ Fresh limes, for serving
√ Fresh cilantro leaves, for serving
√ Sliced cucumber, for serving

DIRECTIONS

1. Combine all of the marinade ingredients together in a large bowl. Whisk to combine thoroughly, then add the chicken. Let marinate for at least 4 hours or overnight.

2. Place the wooden skewers in water and submerge for at least 30 minutes prior to cooking.

3. Whisk together the peanut sauce ingredients in a medium bowl, adding water as needed to thin it out, then set aside.

4. Preheat the Cosori Air Fryer to 380 F.

5. Thread 4-6 pieces of chicken onto each skewer. Place a single layer of skewers in the air fryer basket - you will need to work in batches.

6. Set the air fryer temperature to 380 F and set the timer to 12 minutes. Press Start. Continue to cook the skewers in batches until completed.

7. Serve the chicken satay skewers warm with a side of the peanut sauce, lime wedges, sliced cucumber, and cilantro leaves.

Crispy Spiced Chickpeas

Cooking Time: 17 minutes   Servings: 4

INGREDIENTS

√ 1 (15 ounce) can chickpeas, drained, rinsed, and patted dry
√ 1 tablespoon olive oil
√ ½ teaspoon cumin
√ ¼ teaspoon paprika
√ ½ teaspoon ground fennel seeds
√ ⅛ teaspoon cayenne pepper

DIRECTIONS

1. Combine all ingredients in a large bowl and stir to combine.

2. Select the Preheat function on the Cosori Smart Air Fryer Toaster Oven, adjust temperature to 430°F, and press Start/Pause.

3. Place chickpeas on the food tray, then insert the tray at mid position in the preheated oven.

4. Select the Air Fry function, adjust time to 12 minutes, and press Start/Pause.

5. Remove when chickpeas are crispy and golden.

Air Fried Egg Rolls

Cooking Time: 104 minutes   Servings: 16

INGREDIENTS

√ 1 pound ground pork (70/30)
√ 4 cloves garlic, grated
√ 2 scallions, finely chopped
√ 4-inch piece ginger, peeled and grated
√ 2 tablespoons soy sauce
√ 1 tablespoon sake
√ 1 teaspoon sesame oil
√ 1 cup napa cabbage, finely chopped
√ 4 shiitake mushrooms, stemmed and finely chopped
√ Egg roll wrappers
√ Water
√ Cooking spray

DIRECTIONS

1. Combine ground pork, garlic, scallions, ginger, soy sauce, sake, sesame oil, and napa cabbage, and mushrooms in a large mixing bowl.

2. Mix with a fork making sure not to overmix, until ingredients are evenly distributed.

3. Cover the meat directly with plastic wrap and place in the fridge for 1 hour.

4. Separate the meat into 16 equal portions and roll them into 4 inch longs

5. Position the egg roll wrapper in a diamond position facing you and place each portion of meat into the back end of the wrapper leaving a 1-inch border.

6. Fold the sides of the wrapper inward, fold the back and over, then tightly roll the wrapper forward.

7. Toward the end of the wrapper use your fingers to dab water on the wrapper to help it seal

8. Spray the egg rolls on each side liberally with cooking spray

9. Select the Preheat function on the Cosori Air Fryer, adjust to 340°F, and press Start/Pause.

10. Adjust the temperature to 340°F, set time to 24 minutes, and press Start/Pause.

11. Flip the egg rolls halfway through cooking and spray lightly with more cooking spray.

12. Serve with sweet chili sauce.

Spam Musubi

INGREDIENTS

√ 2 cups uncooked short-grain white rice
√ 2 cups water
√ 6 tablespoons rice vinegar
√ 2 teaspoons toasted sesame seeds
√ 1 can (12-ounce) spam
√ ¼ cup soy sauce
√ ¼ cup oyster sauce
√ ½ cup sugar
√ Roasted nori sheets, cut into thirds (can substitute for packaged roasted seaweed)

DIRECTIONS

1. Soak rice in water fully submerged for 4 hours. Drain, rinse and set aside.
2. Bring 2 cups of water to a boil on high heat, about 5 minutes.
3. Add the rice to the boiling water and stir.
4. Reduce the heat to a simmer, cover, and cook for 20 minutes.
5. Remove the rice when done cooking into a bowl.
6. Distribute the vinegar evenly through the rice by pouring the vinegar over a rice scoop over the rice. Mix gently and set aside to cool.
7. Slice the spam into 8 even slices. Set aside and save the can.
8. Mix together soy sauce, oyster sauce, and sugar in a microwave safe bowl.
9. Microwave for 1 minute and stir, making sure all the sugar is dissolved.
10. Place the spam in the soy sauce mixture and marinate for 10 minutes.
11. Select the Preheat function on the Cosori Air Fryer, adjust to 380°F, then press Start/Pause.
12. Place the spam in the preheated air fryer basket.
13. Cook at 380°F for 6 minutes.
14. Remove the spam from the air fryer and set aside.
15. Line plastic wrap inside of the spam can, covering the whole inside of the can leaving 1 inch or more of plastic wrap on the outside.
16. Place the cooked rice in the plastic wrapped lined spam can about 1¾ inches tall, with one slice of spam on top of the rice, then fold the plastic wrap inside the can pressing down firmly.
17. Remove the spam musubi from the can and remove the plastic. Repeat this process with the remaining spam musubi.
18. Wrap the musubis with roasted nori sheets with the ends of the sheets ending on the bottom. The rice should still be warm. If you microwave for a few seconds.

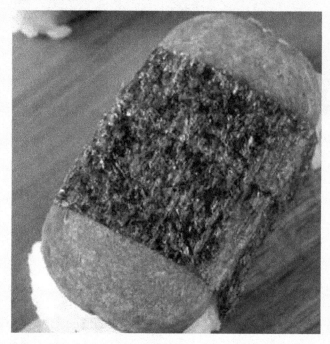

Yogurt Chicken Skewers

Cooking Time: 260 minutes   Servings: 2-4

INGREDIENTS

√ ½ cup plain whole milk Greek yogurt
√ 1 tablespoon olive oil
√ 1 teaspoon paprika
√ ¼ teaspoon cumin
√ ½ teaspoon crushed red pepper
√ 2 wooden skewers, halved
√ 1 lemon, juiced & zested
√ 1 teaspoon salt
√ ¼ teaspoon freshly ground black pepper
√ 4 garlic cloves, minced
√ 1 pound chicken thighs, boneless, skinless, cut into 1½-inch pieces
√ Cooking Spray

DIRECTIONS

1. MIX together the yogurt, olive oil, paprika, cumin, red pepper, lemon juice, lemon zest, salt, pepper, and garlic in a large bowl.
2. ADD the chicken to the marinade and marinate in the fridge for at least 4 hours.
3. SELECT Preheat and press Start/Pause.
4. CUT the marinated chicken thighs into 1½-inch pieces and skewer them onto the halved skewers.
5. PLACE skewers into the preheated air fryer and spray with cooking spray.
6. COOK at 400°F for 10 minutes.

Scotch Egg

Cooking Time: 25 minutes   Servings: 4

INGREDIENTS

√ 10 ounces ground pork sausage
√ ½ teaspoon garlic powder
√ ½ teaspoon onion powder
√ ½ teaspoon dried sage
√ ½ teaspoon salt
√ Cooking spray
√ ¼ teaspoon black pepper
√ 4 eggs, soft boiled, peeled
√ ½ cup all-purpose flour
√ 1 egg, beaten
√ ¾ cup Italian style breadcrumbs

DIRECTIONS

1. MIX together the sausage, garlic powder, onion powder, sage, salt, and pepper. Divide into four balls.
2. WRAP the sausage around each of the peeled medium boiled eggs until the egg is fully covered.
3. COAT each sausage-covered egg with flour, then dip in beaten egg, and roll in breadcrumbs. Dip in the egg and breadcrumbs again.
4. SELECT Preheat on the Cosori Air Fryer, adjust to 350°F, and press Start/Pause.
5. SPRAY the scotch eggs liberally with cooking spray.
6. PLACE the scotch eggs in the preheated air fryer.
7. SELECT Frozen Foods, adjust time to 15 minutes, and press Start/Pause. Make sure to flip the eggs halfway through cooking (the Shake Reminder function will let you know when!).

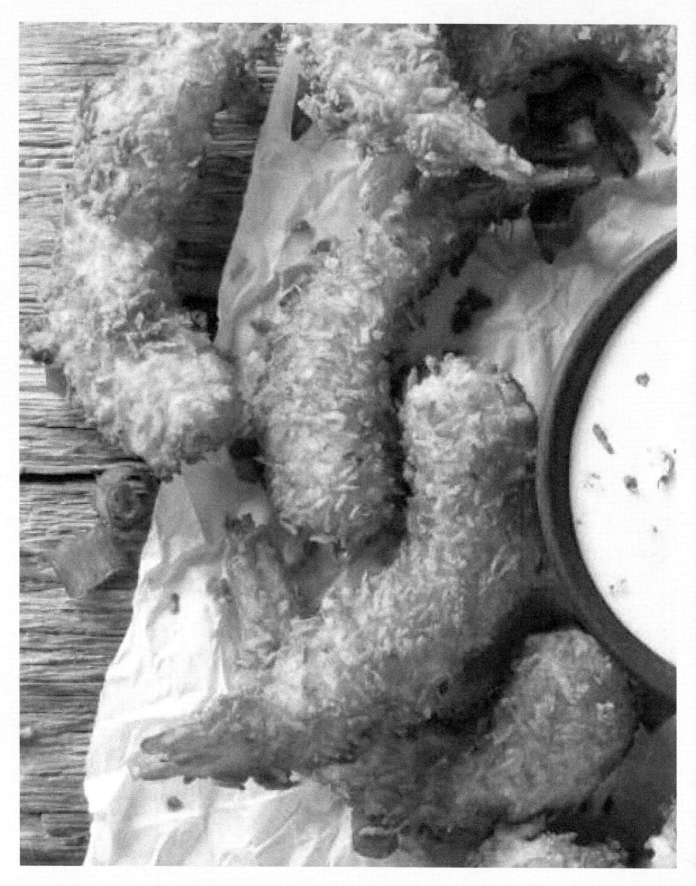

Coconut Shrimp

Cooking Time: 16 minutes   Servings: 3

INGREDIENTS
√ ¼ cup all-purpose flour
√ 1 teaspoon salt, divided
√ ½ teaspoon black pepper, divided
√ ½ teaspoon garlic powder, divided
√ ½ teaspoon paprika, divided
√ 2 large eggs, beaten
√ 1 tablespoon milk
√ ¼ cup panko breadcrumbs
√ ½ cup unsweetened flaked coconut
√ ½ pound large shrimp, peeled (tails left on) & deveined
√ Cooking spray

DIRECTIONS
1. Mix together the flour and half of the seasonings and spices in one bowl. Whisk together the eggs and milk in a separate bowl.
2. Combine the panko breadcrumbs, coconut, and the other half of the seasonings and spices in an additional bowl.
3. Coat each shrimp with flour, then dip in egg, and then roll in breadcrumbs and coconut. Dip in egg and crumbs again. Set aside.
4. Select Preheat on the Cosori Air Fryer, adjust to 350°F, and press Start/Pause.
5. Add the shrimp evenly into the preheated air fryer and spray with Cooking Spray.
6. Select Frozen Foods, adjust time to 8 minutes, and press Start/Pause.
7. Flip the shrimp halfway through cooking (the Shake Reminder function will let you know when!).

Bacon Wrapped Shrimp

Cooking Time: 21 minutes   Servings: 4-5

INGREDIENTS
√ 16 jumbo shrimp, peeled & deveined
√ 1 teaspoon garlic powder
√ 1 teaspoon paprika
√ 1 teaspoon onion powder
√ ¼ teaspoon ground black pepper
√ 8 strips bacon, sliced lengthwise

DIRECTIONS
1. Place the jumbo shrimp in a bowl and season with spices.
2. Wrap the bacon around the shrimp, starting at the top and finishing at the tail, and secure them with toothpicks.
3. Select Preheat on the Cosori Air Fryer, adjust to 320°F, and press Start/Pause.
4. Add half the shrimp to the preheated air fryer.
5. Select Bacon and press Start/Pause. When cooking finishes, set aside.
6. Repeat with the other batch of shrimp.
7. Drain any excess grease on a paper towel and serve.

Bacon-Wrapped Stuffed Jalapeños

Cooking Time: 26 minutes   Servings: 2

INGREDIENTS

√ 6 medium jalapeños, halved lengthwise & deseeded
√ ¼ pound ground pork
√ 2 ounces cheddar cheese
√ Salt & pepper, to taste
√ 6 strips bacon, halved

DIRECTIONS

1. Cut the jalapeños in half, lengthwise, and remove all seeds. Set aside.
2. Combine ground pork, cheddar, salt, and pepper in a bowl and mix until well combined.
3. Spoon about 1 tablespoon of pork mixture into each jalapeño half.
4. Put the jalapeño halves back together and wrap each jalapeño with bacon.
5. Select Preheat on the Cosori Air Fryer, adjust to 320°F, and press Start/Pause.
6. Place the bacon-wrapped jalapeños into the preheated air fryer.
7. Select Bacon, adjust time to 16 minutes, and press Start/Pause.
8. Serve with your favorite dipping sauce.

"Fried" Pickles

Cooking Time: 18 minutes   Servings: 4

INGREDIENTS

√ 4 large dill pickles
√ ½ cup all-purpose flour
√ 2 eggs, beaten
√ ½ cup breadcrumbs
√ 1 teaspoon paprika
√ ⅛ teaspoon cayenne pepper
√ Cooking Spray
√ Salt & pepper, to taste

DIRECTIONS

1. Dry the dill pickles very well with a clean kitchen towel and cut into spears.
2. Set Up a dredging station using 3 shallow bowls. Fill the first shallow dish with flour. Beat the egg in the second dish. Then combine the breadcrumbs, spices, salt and pepper until well incorporated in the last dish.
3. Select Preheat on the Cosori Air Fryer, adjust to 360°F, and press Start/Pause.
4. Coat the pickles by dredging them first in the flour, then the egg, and then the breadcrumbs, pressing the crumbs on gently with your hands. Set the coated pickles on a tray and spray them on all sides with cooking spray.
5. Add the pickles to the preheated air fryer and cook at 360°F for 10 minutes, turning them over halfway through cooking and spraying lightly again, if necessary.
6. Serve with your favorite dipping sauce.

Roasted Garlic & Herb Chicken

Cooking Time: 55 minutes   Servings: 3

INGREDIENTS

√ 3 chicken thighs, bone-in, skin on
√ 3 chicken legs, skin on
√ 2 tablespoons olive oil
√ 2 tablespoons garlic powder
√ 1 teaspoon salt
√ ½ teaspoon black pepper
√ ½ teaspoon dried thyme
√ ½ teaspoon dried rosemary
√ ½ teaspoon dried tarragon

DIRECTIONS

1. Coat the chicken thighs and legs in olive oil and all seasonings. Allow to marinate for 30 minutes.

2. Select Preheat on the Cosori Air Fryer, adjust to 380°F, and press Start/Pause.
3. Place the chicken into the preheated air fryer.
4. Select Chicken, adjust time to 20 minutes, and press Start/Pause.

"Fried" Mozzarella Bites

Cooking Time: 18 minutes   Servings: 3

INGREDIENTS

√ 6 pieces string cheese
√ 2 tablespoons all-purpose flour
√ 1 teaspoon cornstarch
√ ½ teaspoon salt
√ ¼ teaspoon black pepper
√ 2 eggs, beaten
√ 1 tablespoon milk
√ 1 teaspoon dried parsley flakes
√ Cooking Spray
√ Marinara sauce or ranch, for serving

DIRECTIONS

1. CUT the string cheese into thirds, making 18 pieces.
2. MIX together the flour, cornstarch, salt, and pepper in a bowl. Whisk together the eggs and milk in a separate bowl. Combine the panko breadcrumbs and parsley flakes in an additional bowl.
3. COAT each piece of cheese with flour, then dip in egg, and then roll in breadcrumbs. Dip in egg and breadcrumbs again.
4. SELECT Preheat on the Cosori Air Fryer, adjust to 350°F, and press Start/Pause.
5. SET the mozzarella bites in the freezer while the air fryer is preheating.
6. PLACE the coated mozzarella bites into the preheated air fryer and spray liberally with cooking spray.
7. SELECT Frozen Foods, set time for 8 minutes, and press Start/Pause.
8. SHAKE the baskets halfway through cooking (the Shake Reminder function will let you know when!).
9. SERVE with a side of your favorite marinara sauce, or even better, ranch.

Pesto & Sundried Tomato Pinwheels

Cooking Time: 75minutes   Servings: 20

INGREDIENTS
√ 2 sheets pre-made puff pastry, thawed
√ ½ cup pesto sauce
√ 1½ cups mozzarella cheese, shredded, divided
√ ½ cup sundried tomatoes, finely chopped

DIRECTIONS
1. Roll out both puff pastry sheets into 13 x 13-inch squares.
2. Spread the pesto sauce on the first puff pastry sheet. Sprinkle with ½ cup shredded mozzarella.
3. Roll the puff pastry into a log, finishing with the seam side down.
4. Cut into 1-inch-thick pieces.
5. Select the Preheat function on the Cosori Air Fryer, set temperature to 300°F, then press Start/Pause.
6. Line the preheated inner basket with parchment paper, then place the puff pastry pieces on top spiral-side up. You may have to work in batches.
7. Insert the baskets into the preheated air fryer, set time to 25 minutes, then press Start/Pause.
8. Remove baskets when done, flip pinwheels over, then cook for another 5 minutes.
9. Remove when pinwheels are golden brown.
10. Spread the sundried tomatoes and remaining 1 cup shredded mozzarella on the second puff pastry sheet.
11. Repeat steps 3-9, then serve.

Sausage-Stuffed Mushrooms

Cooking Time: 28 minutes   Servings: 3

INGREDIENTS
√ 6 extra-large crimini mushrooms
√ 3 tablespoons olive oil, divided
√ ¼ large onion, diced
√ 1 garlic clove, minced
√ 4 ounces sweet Italian sausage, casing removed
√ 2 tablespoons Italian style breadcrumbs
√ ½ cup mozzarella cheese, shredded, plus more for topping
√ ¼ cup Parmesan cheese, grated
√ 1 tablespoon parsley, freshly chopped
√ Salt & pepper, to taste

DIRECTIONS
1. REMOVE the mushroom stems from the caps. Mince the stems and set aside.
2. SPOON out the insides of the mushroom caps to create more room for the stuffing. Set aside.
3. HEAT a pan on medium-high heat and allow to heat up.
4. ADD 1 tablespoon olive oil, minced mushrooms stems, and diced onions. Cook for 5 minutes.
5. ADD the garlic and cook for 1 minute.
6. ADD in the Italian sausage and cook until brown, about 5 minutes. Set aside.
7. MIX the sausage with the breadcrumbs, mozzarella, Parmesan, and parsley.
8. SEASON to taste with salt and pepper.
9. STUFF the mushrooms until full and top with more mozzarella cheese.
10. DRIZZLE the rest of the oil on the mushrooms.
11. SELECT Preheat on the Cosori Air Fryer, adjust to 320°F, and allow to heat up.
12. PLACE the stuffed mushrooms into the preheated air fryer.
13. COOK the mushrooms at 320°F for 12 minutes until cheese is golden brown and bubbly.

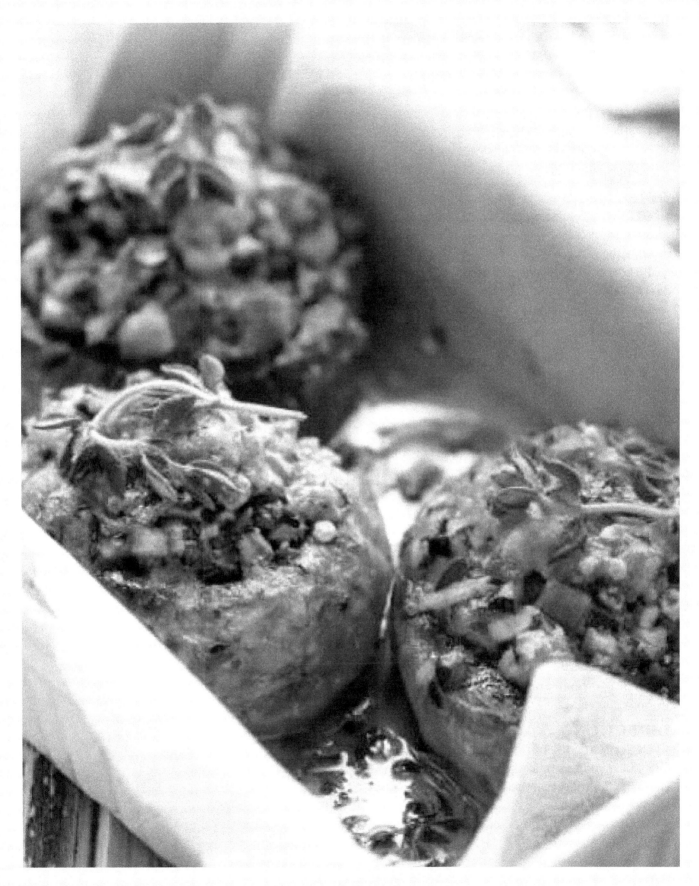

Pigs in a Blanket

Cooking Time: 15 minutes   Servings: 4

INGREDIENTS

√ ½ sheet puff pastry, thawed
√ 16 cocktail-size smoked link sausages
√ 1 tablespoon milk

DIRECTIONS

1. SELECT Preheat on the Cosori Air Fryer and press Start/Pause.
2. CUT the puff pastry into 2½ x 1½-inch strips.
3. PLACE a cocktail sausage on one end of the puff pastry and wrap the dough around the sausage, sealing the dough together with some water.
4. BRUSH the upside (seam-side down) of the wrapped sausages with milk and place in the preheated air fryer.
5. COOK at 400°F for 10 minutes, or until golden brown.

Homemade Tortilla Chips

Cooking Time: 10 minutes   Servings: 2-3

INGREDIENTS

√ 3 corn tortillas (6-inch), cut into 8 pieces each
√ ½ teaspoon salt
√ 1 tablespoon olive oil
√ Salsa, for serving

DIRECTIONS

1. CUT the tortillas in half, then each half into quarters, making a total of 8 pieces per tortilla.
2. SELECT Preheat on the Cosori Air Fryer, adjust to 300°F, and press Start/Pause.
3. TOSS the tortillas in the olive oil and salt until all the chips are well coated.
4. PLACE the tortillas chips in the preheated air fryer and cook for 8 minutes at 300°F.
5. SHAKE the baskets halfway through cooking.
6. SERVE with salsa.

Jerk Chicken Wings

Cooking Time: 30 minutes   Servings: 2-3

INGREDIENTS
√ 2 teaspoons ground thyme
√ 2 teaspoons dried rosemary
√ 2 teaspoons allspice
√ 2 teaspoons ground ginger
√ 1 teaspoon garlic powder
√ 1/3 teaspoon salt
√ 1-2 pounds chicken wings
√ 1 teaspoon onion powder
√ 1 teaspoon cinnamon
√ 1 teaspoon paprika
√ 1 teaspoon chili powder
√ ½ teaspoon nutmeg
√ ¼ cup vegetable oil
√ 1 lime, juiced

DIRECTIONS
1. SELECT Preheat on the Cosori Air Fryer, adjust to 380°F, and press Start/Pause.
2. COMBINE all spices and oil together in a bowl to make a marinade.
3. TOSS the chicken wings in the marinade until wings are well coated.
4. PLACE the chicken wings into the preheated air fryer.
5. SELECT Chicken and press Start/Pause. Make sure to shake the baskets halfway through cooking.
6. REMOVE the wings and place on a serving platter.
7. SQUEEZE fresh lime juice over wings and serve.

Garlic Parmesan Chicken Wings

Cooking Time: 30 minutes   Servings: 3

INGREDIENTS
√ 2 tablespoons cornstarch
√ 4 tablespoons Parmesan, grated
√ 1 tablespoon garlic powder
√ Salt & pepper, to taste
√ 1½ pounds chicken wings
√ Cooking Spray

DIRECTIONS
1. SELECT Preheat on the Cosori Air Fryer, adjust to 380°F, and press Start/Pause.
2. COMBINE the cornstarch, Parmesan, garlic powder, salt, and pepper in a bowl.
3. TOSS the chicken wings into the seasoning and dredge until the wings are well coated.
4. SPRAY the air fryer baskets with cooking spray and add the wings, spraying the top of the chicken wings as well.
5. SELECT Chicken and press Start/Pause. Make sure to shake the baskets halfway through cooking.
6. SPRINKLE with the leftover Parmesan mix and serve.

Honey-Sriracha Wings

Cooking Time: 35 minutes   Servings: 2-4

INGREDIENTS
√ ½ teaspoon smoked paprika
√ ½ teaspoon garlic powder
√ ½ teaspoon onion powder
√ ½ teaspoon salt
√ ¼ teaspoon black pepper
√ 1 tablespoon rice wine vinegar
√ 2 tablespoons cornstarch
√ 1 pound chicken wings
√ Cooking Spray
√ 1/3 cup honey
√ 1/3 cup Sriracha
√ ¼ teaspoon sesame oil

DIRECTIONS
1. SELECT Preheat, adjust to 380°F, and press Start/Pause.
2. MIX together the smoked paprika, garlic powder, onion powder, salt, black pepper, and cornstarch.
3. TOSS the wings in the seasoned cornstarch until all the wings are evenly coated.
4. SPRAY the wings with cooking spray and mix around until all the wings are coated with oil.
5. PLACE the wings in the preheated air fryer.
6. SELECT Chicken, adjust time to 30 minutes, and press Start/Pause.
7. SHAKE the baskets halfway through cooking.
8. WHISK together the honey, Sriracha, rice wine vinegar, and sesame oil in a large bowl.
9. TOSS the cooked wings in the sauce until the are well coated and serve.

Mongolian Chicken Wings

Cooking Time: 40 minutes   Servings: 2-4

INGREDIENTS
√ 1½ pounds chicken wings
√ 1½ tablespoons vegetable oil
√ Salt & pepper, to taste
√ ¼ cup low-sodium soy sauce
√ ¼ cup honey
√ 2 tablespoons rice wine vinegar
√ 1 tablespoon Sriracha
√ 3 garlic cloves, minced
√ 1 tablespoon fresh ginger, grated
√ 1 green onion, chopped, for garnish

DIRECTIONS
1. SELECT Preheat on the Cosori Air Fryer, adjust to 380°F, and press Start/Pause.
2. TOSS chicken wings, oil, salt, and pepper together until well coated.
3. PLACE coated chicken wings into the preheated air fryer.
4. SELECT Chicken and press Start/Pause.
5. COMBINE soy sauce, honey, rice wine vinegar, Sriracha, garlic, and ginger in a saucepan.
6. BRING to a simmer until the flavors meld and the glaze reduces slightly, about 10 minutes.
7. TRANSFER wings, after 20 minutes, into a large bowl and toss with the glaze.
8. RETURN wings to the air fryer baskets and finish cooking for the remaining 5 minutes.
9. GARNISH with green onions and serve.

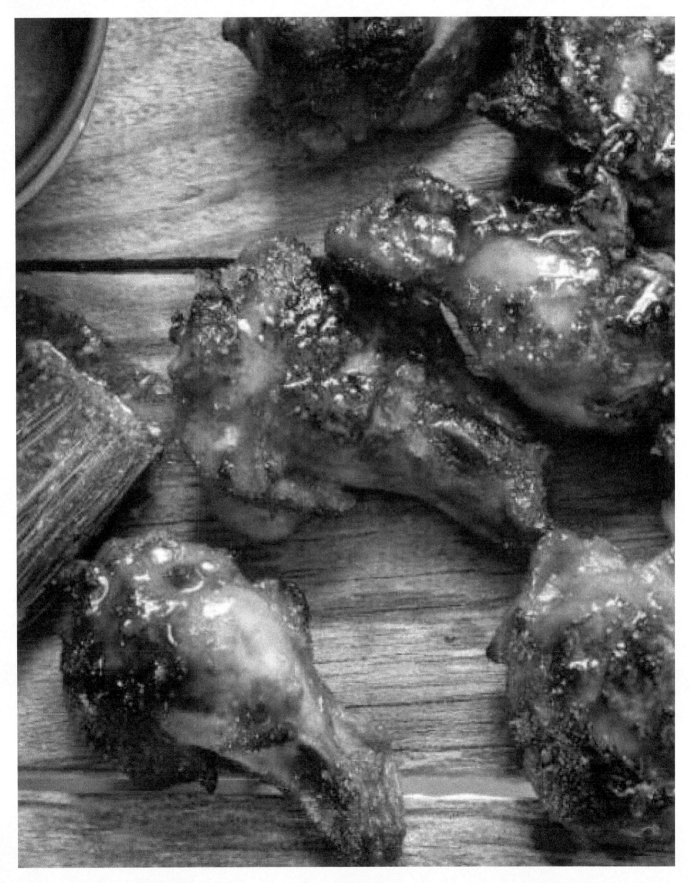

Dry Rubbed Chicken Wings

Cooking Time: 35 minutes   Servings: 4

INGREDIENTS

√ 1 tablespoon granulated garlic
√ 1 chicken bouillon cube, reduced sodium
√ 1 tablespoon salt-free garlic and herb seasoning blend
√ 1 teaspoon salt
√ 1 teaspoon black pepper
√ 1 pound chicken wings
√ Ranch, for serving
√ 1 teaspoon smoked paprika
√ 1 teaspoon cayenne pepper
√ 1 teaspoon Old Bay seasoning, less sodium
√ 1 teaspoon onion powder
√ ½ teaspoon dried oregano
√ Cooking Spray

DIRECTIONS

1. SELECT Preheat on the Cosori Air Fryer, adjust to 380°F, and press Start/Pause.
2. COMBINE seasonings in a bowl and mix well.
3. SEASON the chicken wings with half of the seasoning blend and spray liberally with cooking spray.
4. PLACE the chicken wings into the preheated air fryer.
5. SELECT Chicken, adjust time to 30 minutes, and press Start/Pause.
6. SHAKE the baskets halfway through cooking.
7. TRANSFER the wings into a bowl and sprinkle with the other half of the seasoning until they are well coated.
8. SERVE with a side of ranch.

Lamb Shawarma Skewers

Cooking Time: 20 minutes   Servings: 2

INGREDIENTS

√ ¾ pound ground lamb
√ 1 teaspoon cumin
√ 1 teaspoon paprika
√ 1 teaspoon garlic powder
√ 1 teaspoon onion powder
√ 4 bamboo skewers (9 inches)
√ ½ teaspoon cinnamon
√ ½ teaspoon turmeric
√ ½ teaspoon fennel seeds
√ ½ teaspoon ground coriander seed
√ ½ teaspoon salt

DIRECTIONS

1. COMBINE all ingredients in a bowl and mix well.
2. SKEWER 3 ounces of meat onto each stick, then place in the fridge for 10 minutes.
3. SELECT Preheat on the Cosori Air Fryer and press Start/Pause.
4. PLACE skewers into the preheated air fryer, select Steak, adjust time to 8 minutes, and press Start/Pause.
5. SERVE with lemon yogurt dressing or by itself.

Teriyaki Pork Skewers

Cooking Time: 43 minutes   Servings: 2-4

INGREDIENTS
√ 1 tablespoon cornstarch
√ ½ cup water
√ ¼ cup soy sauce
√ ¼ cup light brown sugar, lightly packed
√ 1 garlic clove, minced
√ Salt & pepper, to taste
√ ½ teaspoon grated ginger
√ Black pepper, to taste
√ 1 pound pork loin chop, cut into 1½-inch cubes
√ 2 wood skewers, halved
√ Cooking Spray

DIRECTIONS
1. WHISK the cornstarch and water together.
2. COMBINE the cornstarch slurry, soy sauce, brown sugar, garlic, and ginger in a small saucepan. Cook the sauce on high heat until it boils and thickens, about 5 minutes.
3. SEASON the sauce to taste with black pepper and allow to cool.
4. SKEWER the pork evenly between the wooden skewers.
5. MARINATE the skewered pork in some of the teriyaki sauce for 30 minutes.
6. SELECT Preheat on the Cosori Air Fryer and press Start/Pause.
7. PLACE the skewers in the preheated air fryer and spray with cooking spray.
8. SELECT Steak, adjust to 8 minutes, and press Start/Pause.
9. BRUSH the skewers with the teriyaki sauce every 2 minutes during cooking.
10. SEASON to taste with salt and pepper, and serve.

Korean Style Beef Skewers

Cooking Time: 71 minutes   Servings: 2-4

INGREDIENTS
√ 1 tablespoon ssamjang
√ 1 tablespoon gochujang
√ 1 tablespoon soy sauce
√ 1 tablespoon sesame oil
√ 1 tablespoon honey
√ 1 teaspoon rice wine vinegar
√ 1 pound beef flap meat, cut into 1½-inch pieces
√ 2 wooden skewers, halved

DIRECTIONS
1. MIX the ssamjang, gochujang, soy sauce, sesame oil, honey, and vinegar in a bowl.
2. TOSS the cut beef into the marinade and marinate for 1 hour.
3. SELECT Preheat on the Cosori Air Fryer and press Start/Pause.
4. SKEWER the pieces of beef onto the halved skewers and place the skewers into the preheated air fryer.
5. SELECT Steak and press Start/Pause.

MEAT RECIPES

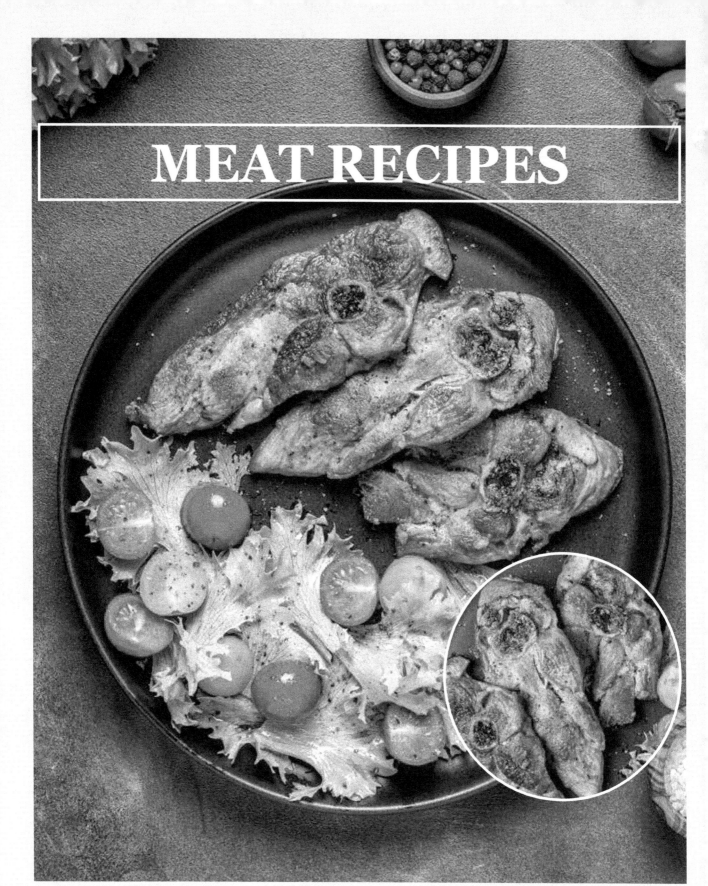

Duxelles Stuffed Pork Loin

INGREDIENTS

Duxelles Stuffing:
√ 1 tablespoon extra virgin olive oil
√ 4 ounces shallots, minced
√ 1 pound baby bella mushrooms, stems removed and minced
√ Kosher salt, to taste
√ Black pepper, to taste
√ 3 tablespoons Parmesan cheese, grated
√ ¼ cup Pecorino Romano cheese, grated
√ 1/3 cup panko breadcrumbs

Pork Loin:
√ 2 cuts pork loin (5 ounces each)
√ 2 tomatoes, diced, liquid reserved
√ Kosher salt, for seasoning
√ Black pepper, for seasoning
√ 2 tablespoons unsalted butter
√ 2 sprigs rosemary
√ 4 cloves garlic, smashed
√ Oil spray
√ 1 can marinara sauce (16 ounces), warmed
√ 2 tablespoons parsley, roughly chopped, for serving

DIRECTIONS

Duxelles Stuffing:
1. Heat a large sauté pan over medium heat and lightly coat the pan with olive oil.
2. Add the shallots and sauté until translucent, about 5 minutes. Then, add the mushrooms and let them cook until all the water is released and evaporates.
3. Season to taste with salt and pepper, then remove from heat.
4. Combine the mushroom mixture with the Parmesan cheese, Pecorino Romano cheese, and panko breadcrumbs in a medium bowl. Season to taste with salt and pepper, then set aside.

Pork Loin:
5. Place the pork loins into a large bowl with the diced tomatoes and liquid. Cover and let sit in the refrigerator for 15 minutes.
6. Remove the pork loins from the diced tomatoes and pat dry.
7. Trim any excess fat from the loins, then, using a paring knife, cut out a ¾-inch circle completely through each pork loin.
8. Stuff the pork loin with the duxelles, packing in the stuffing firmly. Using your hands, flatten both sides of each loin to ensure the hole is filled and leveled with the meat.
9. Season the loins lightly with salt and pepper.
10. Place a medium sauté pan over high heat. Add the butter and melt completely. Add the rosemary and garlic and heat until aromatic, about 3 minutes.
11. Sear pork loin on both sides until golden, about 2 minutes on each side, then immediately remove from heat and set aside.
12. Select the Preheat function on the Cosori Air Fryer, adjust temperature to 350°F, and press Start/Pause.
13. Spray the inner air fryer basket with oil spray, then place the pork into the preheated air fryer.
14. Set temperature to 350°F and time to 12 minutes, press Shake, then press Start/Pause.
Note: Cooking time may vary on thickness of cut. For a cut 1-2 inches thick, cooking time will take 10 to 12 minutes.
15. Flip the pork loins halfway through cooking. The Shake Reminder will let you know when.
16. Remove the pork loins when done and rest for 5 minutes.
17. Assemble the stuffed pork loins by placing 3 ounces of marina sauce on the plate, placing the pork loins on top, and sprinkling with parsley.
18. Serve immediately, with extra marinara sauce on the side if desired.

Juicy Lucy Sliders

INGREDIENTS

Burger Patties:
- √ 1 pound ground beef
- √ 1½ teaspoons kosher salt
- √ 1 tablespoon ground black pepper
- √ 1 tablespoon onion powder
- √ 6 slices American cheese
- √ Oil spray

For Serving:
- √ 6 slider buns, sliced in half & toasted
- √ Ketchup
- √ Mustard
- √ Mayonnaise
- √ Lettuce
- √ Tomato
- √ Onion

DIRECTIONS

1. Combine the ground beef, salt, pepper, and onion powder in a large bowl.
2. Divide the meat into 6 equal portions.
3. Form a patty with each portion, then press the cheese into the center of each until the cheese is completely enclosed by the meat. Set aside.
4. Select the Preheat function on the Cosori Air Fryer, adjust temperature to 380°F, then press Start/Pause.
5. Spray the preheated air fryer basket with oil spray.
6. Place the burger patties into the preheated air fryer.
7. Set temperature to 380°F and time to 14 minutes, press Shake, then press Start/Pause.
8. Flip the burger patties halfway through cooking. The Shake Reminder will let you know when.
9. Remove the burger patties when done and let rest for 5 minutes.
10. Assemble the burgers with toasted buns, ketchup, mustard, mayonnaise, lettuce, tomato, and onion.
11. Serve the sliders warm.

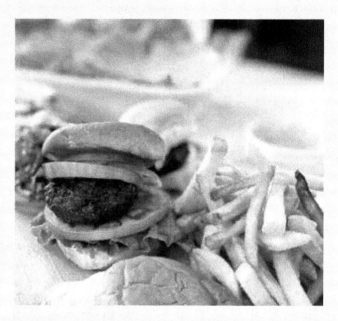

Barbecue Baby Back Ribs

Cooking Time: 35 minutes   Servings: 4

INGREDIENTS
√ 1 rack pork baby back ribs
√ 1½ teaspoons black pepper
√ 1½ teaspoons smoked paprika
√ ½ cup barbecue
√ sauce
√ 2 teaspoons kosher salt
√ 1½ teaspoons garlic powder
√ 1 teaspoon mustard powder

DIRECTIONS
1. Select the Preheat function on the Cosori Air Fryer, adjust temperature to 380°F, and press Start/Pause.
2. Peel the membrane from the back of the ribs by sliding a dinner knife under the membrane and over the bone. Lift and loosen the membrane until it tears, then hold the edge of the membrane with a paper towel to pull it off.
Note: The membrane may come off in one whole piece, or you may need to remove it in smaller pieces.
3. Cut the rack into 3 equal sections, then dry the ribs thoroughly with paper towels.
4. Combine the salt, pepper, garlic powder, smoked paprika, and mustard powder in a small bowl and mix until combined.
5. Season the ribs on both sides with the spice mixture.
6. Wrap each section of ribs tightly with foil, then place the ribs meat-side down into the preheated air fryer basket.
7. Set temperature to 380°F and time to 25 minutes, then press Start/Pause.
8. Remove the ribs when done and carefully unwrap the aluminum foil.
9. Brush the ribs on each side with barbecue sauce, then place them back into the air fryer basket meat-side up.
10. Set temperature to 380°F and time to 10 minutes, then press Start/Pause.
11. Remove the ribs from the air fryer when done and let cool slightly before serving.

Rosemary and Thyme Roast Beef

Cooking Time: 175 minutes   Servings: 6-8

INGREDIENTS
√ 3 pound bottom round roast
√ 2 tablespoons olive oil
√ 1 tablespoon salt
√ ½ teaspoon black pepper
√ ½ teaspoon garlic powder
√ ½ teaspoon onion powder
√ ½ teaspoon dried rosemary
√ ½ teaspoon dried thyme
√ ¼ teaspoon ground paprika

DIRECTIONS
1. Trim roast of any silverskin or sinew.
2. Rub the roast with olive oil.
3. Season the roast with salt, black pepper, garlic powder, onion powder, dried rosemary, dried thyme, and paprika.
4. Truss the roast with butcher's twine so it holds it shape.
5. Allow to rest at room temperature for 2 hours.
6. Preheat the air fryer at 330°F for 5 minutes.
7. Place the roast in the preheated air fryer basket.
8. Cook at 330°F for 45 minutes, flipping halfway through cooking.
9. Remove the meat when done coking and allow to rest for 20 minutes.
10. Remove the butcher's twine, slice, and serve.

Bone-in Ribeye with Lemon Chimichurri

Cooking Time: 73 minutes   Servings: 1-2

INGREDIENTS
√ ½ cup firmly packed fresh Italian flat-leaf parsley, destemmed
√ 2 garlic cloves, minced
√ 1 tablespoon fresh oregano leaves, finely chopped
√ 3 tablespoons extra-virgin olive oil
√ 2 tablespoons lemon juice
√ 1 lemon zested
√ ¼ teaspoon crushed red pepper
√ Salt and pepper, to taste
√ 1 (1 pound) bone-in ribeye, 1-inch thick
√ ½ teaspoon salt
√ ¼ teaspoon black pepper

DIRECTIONS
1. Combine parsley, garlic, oregano, olive oil, lemon juice, lemon zest, and crushed red pepper in a mixing bowl.
2. Season the chimichurri to taste with salt and pepper. Set aside.
3. Remove the steak from the fridge and allow it to come to room temperature for 1 hour.
4. Dry the steak with paper towels to remove any moisture.
5. Season the steak with salt and pepper. Set aside.
6. Preheat the air fryer to 400°F for 6 minutes.
7. Place the steak in the preheated air fryer.
8. Cook at 400°F for 8 minutes.
9. Allow the meat to rest for 10 minutes before slicing.
10. Serve with lemon chimichurri.

Montreal Ribeye

Cooking Time: 14 minutes   Servings: 1

INGREDIENTS
√ 1 teaspoon crushed black pepper
√ 1 teaspoon garlic powder
√ 1 teaspoon kosher salt
√ 1 teaspoon paprika
√ ½ teaspoon onion powder
√ ½ teaspoon ground coriander
√ ½ teaspoon dried dill
√ ½ teaspoon crushed red pepper flakes
√ 1 (1 pound) boneless ribeye

DIRECTIONS
1. Mix together the seasoning until well combined.
2. Season the steak on all sides with the seasoning blend.
3. Select Preheat on the Cosori Air Fryer, adjust to 400°F then press Start/Pause.
4. Place seasoned steak into the preheated air fryer basket.
5. Select Steak, set time to 12 minutes, then press Start/Pause.
6. Remove the steak from the air fryer basket and allow the meat to rest for 5 minutes.
7. Slice the steak against the grain after resting.

Red Thai Curry Ribeye

Cooking Time: 259 minutes   Servings: 1

INGREDIENTS
√ 1 (16 oz) boneless rib
√ 1 (4 oz) jar red curry paste
√ ½ (14 oz) can lite coconut milk
√ 1 lime, zested
√ ½ lime juiced
√ 1 tablespoon sugar
√ 1 tablespoon fish sauce
√ ¾ teaspoon salt
√ ¼ teaspoon black pepper

DIRECTIONS
1. Combine all ingredients in a ziplock bag, mix, and marinate in the fridge for 4 hours.
2. Preheat on the Cosori Air Fryer at 400°F for 6 minutes.
3. Wipe off any residual marinade from the steak and set aside.
4. Place marinated steak into the air fryer basket.
5. Set the temperature to 400°F for 14 minutes and press start/stop.
6. Rest the meat for 5 minutes, before slicing.
7. Serve immediately.

Filipino Pork BBQ Skewers

Cooking Time: 27 minutes   Servings: 8

INGREDIENTS
Marinade
√ 1/3 cup light brown sugar, lightly packed
√ ¼ cup soy sauce
√ ¼ cup coconut vinegar
√ 2 tablespoons banana ketchup
√ 6 garlic cloves, grated
√ 1 teaspoons freshly ground black pepper
√ ½ (8 ounce) can lemon lime soda
√ 2 pounds pork shoulder, cut into 1½-inch pieces

Basting Sauce
√ ½ cup used marinade
√ ¼ cup ketchup
√ 2 tablespoons olive oil

DIRECTIONS
1. Mix together all the marinade ingredients in a large bowl, massaging the meat until well combined
2. Cover the bowl with plastic wrap and refrigerate for at least 4 hours.
3. Remove the meat from the fridge and skewer the meat. Set aside.
4. Combine the basting sauce ingredients and microwave for 30 seconds. Set aside.
5. Select the Preheat function on the Cosori Air Fryer and press Start/Pause.
6. Place the meat skewers in the preheated air fryer basket.
7. Select the Steak function, adjust time to 12 minutes, and press Start/Pause.
8. Baste the skewers three times throughout the cooking process.

Turkey Lasagna with Zucchini "Noodles"

Cooking Time: 60 minutes   Servings: 6

INGREDIENTS

√ 1 tbsp olive oil
√ 1 lb ground turkey
√ 1 medium yellow onion, small diced
√ 3 cloves garlic, minced
√ 2 tbsp tomato paste
√ 1 14 oz can tomato puree
√ 1 tbsp chopped fresh oregano (or 1 tsp dried oregano)
√ 1 tbsp chopped fresh thyme leaves (or 1 tsp dried thyme)
√ Kosher salt, as needed
√ ¼ cup torn fresh basil leaves
√ 1 whole egg
√ 6 oz ricotta cheese
√ ½ cup grated parmesan cheese
√ 2 cups mozzarella cheese, freshly grated
√ 2 zucchini, thinly sliced lengthwise

DIRECTIONS

1. Heat a large skillet over medium high. Add the olive oil, and then add the ground turkey. Sprinkle the turkey with salt and then cook until browned, breaking the turkey apart with a spoon as it cooks. After it is browned, push the turkey to the side of the pan.

2. Add the onion to the empty side and cook until translucent. Add the garlic and cook 1 minute longer, then stir in the tomato paste. Coat the turkey mixture with the tomato paste and cook, stirring constantly, until the tomato paste has gone from red to a coppery tone.

3. Pour the tomato puree and herbs into the turkey mixture and simmer for 15-20 minutes over low heat, stirring occasionally. Season with kosher salt to taste, then turn off the heat and set aside.

4. Combine the ricotta, egg, basil, parmesan, and big pinch of salt and black pepper in a bowl and whisk to combine. Set aside.

5. Select Preheat on the Cosori Air Fryer and press Start.

6. Build the lasagna. Spray the inside of the cake pan accessory or a baking dish that will fit inside the Air Fryer basket with olive oil. Spoon a bit of the meat sauce on the very bottom of the pan, then lay 3 slices of zucchini down, and then spread some of the ricotta mixture over the zucchini. Spoon some of the meat sauce over the top of the ricotta, and then top with shredded mozzarella. Repeat these steps until the baking dish is full, ending with extra shredded mozzarella on top. Sprinkle the top with a bit more parmesan cheese. Tightly cover the top of the pan with aluminum foil.

7. Insert the lasagna into the Air Fryer basket. Set the temperature to 350 and set the time to 25 minutes. Remove the foil from the top, set the temperature to 400 and cook 5 minutes more to brown the top. Let cool slightly before serving, then sprinkle with extra fresh basil and thyme.

Chili Lime Beef Skewers

Cooking Time: 130 minutes   Servings: 2

INGREDIENTS

√ 1 (1 pound) ribeye steak, cut in 2 inch cubes
√ ¼ cup olive oil
√ 1 tablespoon chili powder
√ 2 teaspoons salt
√ 1 teaspoon cumin
√ 1 teaspoon oregano
√ ½ teaspoon garlic powder
√ ½ teaspoon black pepper
√ 1 lime, juiced
√ 1 red bell pepper, cut in 2 inch pieces
√ ½ onion, cut in 2 inch pieces

DIRECTIONS

1. Combine steak, olive oil, chili powder, salt, cumin, oregano, black pepper, and lime juice in a Ziploc bag. Shake well.

2. Marinate for 2 hours.

3. Skewer the meat interchanging between red bell pepper and onion. Set aside.

4. Place the broiler pan on the top rack on the Cosori Toaster Oven.

5. Select Broil and adjust time to 10 minutes, then press Start/Cancel to preheat the Cosori Toaster Oven.

6. Place the skewers on the broil pan in preheated toaster oven and then press Start/Cancel

7. Remove the skewers carefully when done, and serve.

Japanese Meatballs

Cooking Time: 25 minutes   Servings: 1

INGREDIENTS

√ 1 pound ground beef
√ 1 tablespoon sesame oil
√ 1 tablespoon Awase miso paste
√ 10 fresh mint leaves, finely chopped
√ 4 scallions, finely chopped
√ 1 teaspoon salt
√ ½ teaspoon black pepper
√ 3 tablespoons soy sauce
√ 3 tablespoons mirin
√ 1 tablespoon water
√ 1 teaspoon brown sugar

DIRECTIONS

1. MIX together the ground beef, sesame oil, miso paste, mint leaves, scallions, salt, and pepper until everything is well incorporated.

2. ADD a small amount of sesame oil to your hands and form mixture into 2-inch meatballs. You should have about 8 meatballs.

3. ALLOW the meatballs to set in the fridge for 10 minutes.

4. CREATE the dipping sauce by mixing together the soy sauce, mirin, water, and brown sugar. Set aside.

5. SELECT Preheat on the Cosori Air Fryer and press Start/Pause.

6. ARRANGE the chilled meatballs in the preheated air fryer.

7. SELECT Steak, adjust time to 10 minutes, and press Start/Pause.

8. SERVE the meatballs with the dipping sauce.

Pork Belly Scallion Yakitori

Cooking Time: 169 minutes   Servings: 3

INGREDIENTS

√ ¼ cup soy sauce

√ 1 tablespoon sake

√ 2 tablespoons mirin

√ 2 teaspoons rice wine vinegar

√ 2 teaspoons sugar

√ 2 tablespoons dark brown sugar

√ ½ teaspoon onion powder

√ ¼ teaspoon garlic powder

√ ¼ teaspoon kosher salt

√ 1½ inch piece of ginger, peeled and roughly sliced

√ 1 pound of ½-inch thick sliced pork belly, cut into 2-inch pieces

√ 6 scallions

√ Lemon wedges, for serving

DIRECTIONS

1. Combine soy sauce, sake, mirin, rice wine vinegar, dark brown sugar, onion powder, garlic powder, kosher salt, and ginger in a bowl.

2. Add the pork belly to the marinade and massage the marinade into the meat.

3. Cover and place into the refrigerator for 5 hours.

4. Remove from the fridge and pat the pork belly dry with paper towels. Set aside and allow to sit at room temperature for 1 hour.

5. Cut off the thinner dark green part of the scallion and discard.

6. Cut the trimmed scallions into thirds.

7. Skewer a piece of pork belly, followed by a piece of scallion, then repeat until the skewer is filled. Place the skewers onto the food tray.

8. Select the Preheat function on the Cosori Smart Air Fryer Toaster Oven, adjust temperature to 450°F, and press Start/Pause.

9. Insert the food tray with yakitori at top position in the preheated oven.

10. Select the Broil and Shake functions, then press Start/Pause.

11. Flip the yakitori halfway through cooking. The Shake Reminder will let you know when.

12. Remove when done and serve with a wedge of lemon.

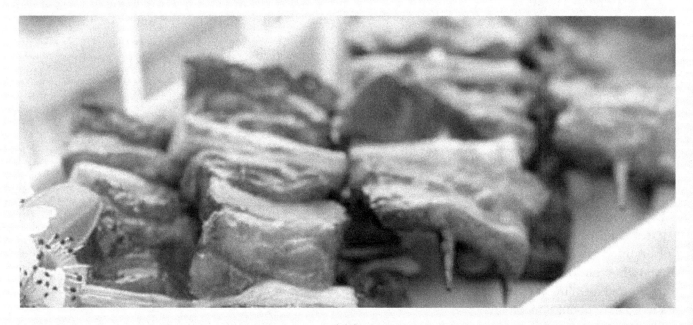

INGREDIENTS

Dough

√ ¾ cup plus 1½ tablespoons warm water, 100°-110°F

√ 1¾ teaspoons instant yeast

√ 2 cups all-purpose flour, plus more for dusting

√ 1 teaspoon kosher salt

√ 1 tablespoon extra virgin olive oil, plus more for drizzling

Toppings

√ 6 tablespoons pizza sauce

√ 8 ounces shredded low-moisture mozzarella

√ Pepperoni slices

√ 8 ounces cooked Italian sausage

√ Crushed red pepper, for sprinkling

√ Dried oregano, for sprinkling

√ Black pepper, for sprinkling

DIRECTIONS

1. Pour water into a large mixing bowl, then whisk in the yeast. Allow to bloom for 10 minutes.

2. Add the flour and salt and mix with your hands until no dry flour remains.

3. Cover the dough tightly with plastic wrap and allow to rest at room temperature for 15 hours.

4. Add the olive oil and form into a ball.

5. Drizzle extra-virgin olive oil generously on the food tray and use your hands to coat evenly.

6. Place the dough on the food tray and spread it out slightly toward the corners of the pan.

7. Drizzle some more extra-virgin olive oil on top and use your hands to evenly coat the top of the dough.

8. Cover the dough and allow it to rest for 90 minutes.

9. Spread the dough out further so that it covers the bottom of the pan, then pop any bubbles that formed in the dough.

10. Spread pizza sauce on the dough, followed by cheese, then pepperoni and sausage.

11. Sprinkle the pizza with crushed red pepper, dried oregano, and black pepper.

12. Select the Preheat function on the Cosori Smart Air Fryer Toaster Oven, adjust temperature to 450°F, and press Start/Pause.

13. Insert the pizza at low position in the preheated oven.

14. Select the Pizza function, adjust time to 15 minutes, and press Start/Pause.

15. Remove when done and allow to rest for 5 minutes before cutting.

16. Cut the pizza into squares and serve.

Beef Bourguignon

Cooking Time: 285 minutes   Servings: 6

INGREDIENTS

√ 4 slices bacon, chopped into ½-inch pieces
√ 3 pounds chuck roast, cut into 2-inch chunks
√ 1 tablespoon kosher salt, plus more to taste
√ 4 tablespoons all purpose flour, divided
√ 4 tablespoons all purpose flour, divided
√ 2 tablespoons olive oil
√ 2 large carrots, cut into ½-inch thick slices
√ ½ large white onion, diced
√ 4 cloves garlic, minced
√ 2 tablespoons tomato paste
√ 3 cups red wine (Merlot, Pinot Noir, or Chianti)
√ 2 cups beef stock
√ 1 beef bouillon cube, crushed
√ ½ teaspoon dried thyme
√ ¼ teaspoon dried parsley
√ 2 bay leaves
√ 10 ounces fresh small white or brown mushrooms, quartered
√ 2 tablespoons cornstarch (optional)
√ 2 tablespoons water (optional)

DIRECTIONS

1. Render the bacon in a large pot over medium heat for 5 minutes or until crispy.
2. Drain the bacon and set aside, leaving the bacon fat in the pot.
3. Mix together chuck roast chunks, kosher salt, black pepper, and 2 tablespoons of all purpose flour until well combined.
4. Dredge the beef of any extra flour and sear in the bacon grease for about 4 minutes on each side. It is important not to overcrowd the pot, so you may need to work in batches.
5. Remove the beef when done and set aside with the bacon.
6. Add the olive oil, sliced carrots, and diced onion to the pot. Cook for 5 minutes, then add the garlic and cook for another minute.

7. Add the tomato paste and cook for 1 minute, then mix in the remaining 2 tablespoons of flour and cook on medium low for 4 minutes.
8. Pour in the wine and beef stock, scraping the bottom of the pot to make sure there aren't any bits stuck to the bottom.
9. Add the bacon and seared meat back into the pot, along with the bouillon cube, dried thyme, dried parsley, bay leaves, and mushrooms. Mix well and bring to a light boil.
10. Insert the wire rack at low position in the Cosori Smart Air Fryer Toaster Oven.
11. Cover the pot with foil and place on the rack in the oven. Make sure the foil is secure so it doesn't lift and contact the heating elements.
12. Select the Slow Cook function, adjust time to 4 hours, and press Start/Pause.
13. Remove the pot carefully from the oven when done and place back on the stove.
14. Discard the foil, mix the stew, and season to taste with salt and pepper.
15. Thicken the stew if desired by using a cornstarch slurry of 2 tablespoons cornstarch and 2 tablespoons water. Add half, mix, and bring to a boil, stirring occasionally. If the sauce is still too thin, add the other half of the slurry.

Chicken Breast with Chermoula Sauce

Cooking Time: 30 minutes   Servings: 4

INGREDIENTS

Chicken
- √ 2 boneless skinless chicken breasts
- √ 1 tablespoon olive oil
- √ 1 teaspoon salt
- √ 1 teaspoon pepper

Chermoula
- √ 1 cup fresh cilantro
- √ 1 cup fresh parsley
- √ ¼ cup fresh mint
- √ ½ teaspoon red chili flakes
- √ ½ teaspoon cumin seeds
- √ ½ teaspoon coriander seeds
- √ 3 garlic cloves, peeled
- √ ½ cup extra virgin olive oil
- √ 1 lemon, zested and juiced
- √ ¾ teaspoons smoked paprika
- √ ¾ teaspoons salt

DIRECTIONS

1. Combine all the chermoula sauce ingredients in a blender or food processor. Pulse until smooth. Taste and add salt if needed. Place into a bowl and set aside.

2. Slice the chicken breast in half lengthwise and lightly pound with a meat tenderizer until both halves are about ½-inch thick.

3. Select the Preheat function on the Cosori Smart Air Fryer Toaster Oven, adjust temperature to 430°F, and press Start/Pause.

4. Line the food tray with foil, then place the chicken breasts on the tray. Drizzle chicken with olive oil and season with salt and pepper.

5. Insert the food tray at top position in the preheated oven.

6. Select the Air Fry function, adjust time to 15 minutes, and press Start/Pause.

7. Remove when the chicken breast reaches an internal temperature of 160°F. Allow the chicken to rest for 5 minutes.

8. Brush the chermoula sauce over the chicken, or serve chicken with chermoula sauce on the side.

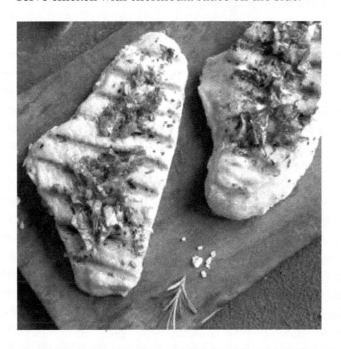

Crab Cakes

INGREDIENTS

Rémoulade
√ ¼ cup mayonnaise
√ 1 teaspoon capers, washed & drained
√ ½ tablespoon sweet pickles, minced
√ ½ tablespoon red onion, finely diced
√ ½ tablespoon lemon juice
√ ½ teaspoon Dijon mustard
√ Salt & pepper, to taste

Crab Cakes
√ 1 large egg, beaten
√ 1¼ tablespoons mayonnaise
√ ¾ teaspoon Dijon mustard
√ 1 teaspoon Worcestershire sauce
√ 1 teaspoon Old Bay seasoning
√ ¼ teaspoon salt
√ A pinch white pepper
√ ¼ cup celery, finely diced
√ ¼ cup red bell pepper, finely diced
√ 2 tablespoons fresh parsley, finely chopped
√ ½ pound lump crab meat
√ 1/3 cup panko breadcrumbs
√ Cooking Spray

DIRECTIONS

1. MIX together rémoulade ingredients until everything is well incorporated. Set aside.
2. WHISK together the egg, mayonnaise, mustard, Worcestershire, Old Bay, salt, white pepper, cayenne pepper, celery, bell pepper, and parsley.
3. GENTLY FLAKE the crab meat into the egg mixture and fold together until well mixed.
4. SPRINKLE the breadcrumbs over the crab mixture and fold gently until breadcrumbs are well incorporated.
5. FORM the crab mixture into 4 cake patties and chill in the fridge for 30 minutes.
6. SELECT Preheat on the Cosori Air Fryer and press Start/Pause.
7. LINE the preheated inner basket with a sheet of parchment paper. Spray the crab cakes with cooking spray and lay them gently onto the paper.
8. COOK the crab cakes at 400°F for 8 minutes until golden brown.
9. FLIP the crab cakes halfway through cooking.
10. SERVE with the rémoulade.

Mediterranean Lamb Meatballs

INGREDIENTS

√ 1 pound ground lamb
√ 3 garlic cloves, minced
√ ¾ teaspoon salt
√ ¼ teaspoon black pepper
√ 1½ tablespoons mint, freshly chopped
√ 1 tablespoon fresh lemon juice
√ 1 teaspoon lemon zest
√ ½ cup breadcrumbs
√ 1 teaspoon ground cumin
√ ½ teaspoon hot sauce
√ ½ teaspoon chili powder
√ 1 scallion, minced
√ 2 tablespoons parsley, finely chopped
√ 1 egg
√ 2 teaspoons olive oil

DIRECTIONS

1. MIX together the lamb, garlic, salt, pepper, mint, cumin, hot sauce, chili powder, scallion, parsley, lemon juice, lemon zest, breadcrumbs, and egg until well combined.
2. FORM the lamb mixture into 9 balls and chill in the fridge for 30 minutes.
3. SELECT Preheat on the Cosori Air Fryer and press Start/Pause.
4. COAT the meatballs in olive oil and place in the preheated air fryer.
5. SELECT Steak, adjust time to 10 minutes, and press Start/Pause.

Italian Meatballs

INGREDIENTS

√ ½ pound ground beef (75/25)
√ ¼ cup panko breadcrumbs
√ ⅛ cup milk
√ 1 egg
√ 1 teaspoon garlic powder
√ Cooking Spray
√ 1 teaspoon onion powder
√ 2 teaspoons dried oregano
√ 1 tablespoon dried parsley
√ Salt & pepper, to taste
√ 3 tablespoons Parmesan cheese, grated, plus more for serving
√ Marinara sauce, for serving

DIRECTIONS

1. COMBINE the ground beef, breadcrumbs, milk, egg, spices, salt, pepper, and Parmesan and mix well.
2. ROLL the meat mixture into medium-sized balls. Set aside in the fridge for 10 minutes.
3. SELECT preheat on the Cosori Air Fryer and press Start/Pause.
4. REMOVE meatballs from the fridge and add to the preheated air fryer baskets. Spray the meatballs with cooking spray and cook at 400F for 8 minutes.
5. SERVE with marinara sauce and more grated Parmesan.

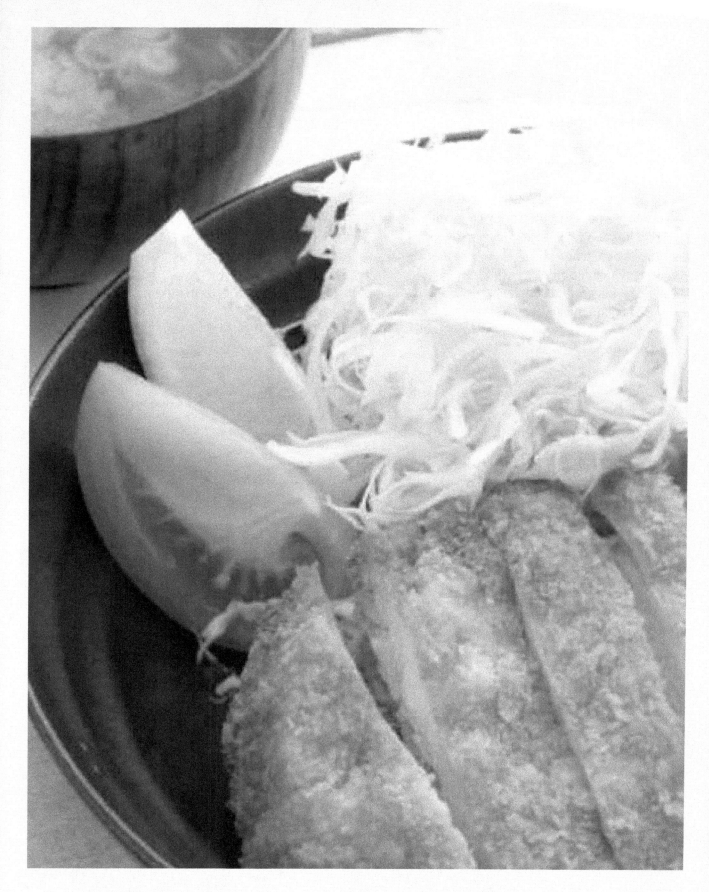

Steak Sandwich

Cooking Time: 11 minutes   Servings: 2

INGREDIENTS

√ 1 ribeye (16 ounces), boneless
√ 1 tablespoon olive oil
√ 1 teaspoon salt
√ ½ teaspoon black pepper
√ ½ cup sour cream
√ 3 tablespoons prepared white horseradish, drained
√ 2 teaspoons chives, freshly chopped
√ 1 small shallot, minced
√ ½ teaspoon lemon juice
√ Salt & pepper, to taste
√ Toasted sesame seed buns, for serving
√ Baby arugula, for serving
√ Shallots, sliced, for serving

DIRECTIONS

1. SELECT Preheat on the Cosori Air Fryer and press Start/Pause.

2. COAT your steak with olive oil and season with the salt and pepper.

3. PLACE the steak into the preheated air fryer.

4. SELECT Steak and press Start/Pause.

5. MIX together the sour cream, horseradish, chives, shallots, and lemon juice in a small bowl.

6. SEASON the horseradish cream with salt and pepper to taste.

7. REMOVE the meat from the air fryer when done cooking, and let rest for 5 to 10 minutes before slicing.

8. ASSEMBLE a sandwich by adding some of the horseradish cream to the bottom bun along with the baby arugula, sliced shallots, and the sliced steak.

Pork Katsu

Cooking Time: 24 minutes   Servings: 2

INGREDIENTS

√ 2 pork chops (6 ounces), boneless
√ ½ cup panko breadcrumbs
√ 1 teaspoon garlic powder
√ 1 teaspoon onion powder
√ 1 teaspoon salt
√ ¼ teaspoon white pepper
√ ½ cup all-purpose flour
√ 2 eggs, beaten
√ Cooking Spray

DIRECTIONS

1. PLACE pork chops into a ziplock bag or cover with plastic wrap.

2. POUND the pork with a rolling pin or meat hammer until it has a ½-inch thickness.

3. COMBINE the breadcrumbs and seasonings in a bowl. Set aside.

4. DREDGE each pork chop in the flour, then dip in the beaten eggs, and roll in the breadcrumb mixture.

5. SELECT Preheat on the Cosori Air Fryer, adjust to 360°F, and press Start/Pause.

6. SPRAY both sides of the pork with cooking spray and place into the preheated air fryer.

7. COOK the pork chops at 360°F for 14 minutes.

8. REMOVE from air fryer when done cooking, and allow to rest for 5 minutes.

9. SLICE into pieces and serve.

Citrus Roasted Chicken

Cooking Time: 55 minutes   Servings: 4

INGREDIENTS

√ 1 3lb whole chicken
√ 1 small lemon, quartered
√ ½ small orange, quartered
√ 1 shallot, peeled and halved
√ 3 garlic cloves, minced
√ 4 thyme sprigs
√ 2 rosemary sprigs
√ 3 tablespoons olive oil
√ 3 tablespoons lemon juice
√ 3 tablespoons orange juice
√ 1 tablespoon honey
√ 1 cup chicken stock
√ 1 teaspoon cornstarch
√ Salt and pepper

DIRECTIONS

1. Pat the chicken dry inside and out. Season well inside and out with salt and pepper. Place the lemon, orange, shallot, thyme, and rosemary in the cavity of the chicken. Tie the legs together with kitchen twine. Brush 1 tablespoon of the olive oil over the chicken.

2. Select the Preheat function on the Cosori Air Fryer, adjust temperature to 360°F, and press Start/Pause.

3. Place chicken breast side down into the preheated air fryer basket. Pour the chicken stock in the bottom of the fryer basket.

4. Set time to 20 minutes, temperature to 360°F, and press Start/Pause.

5. Whisk together the 2 tablespoons of olive oil, lemon juice, orange juice, 3 garlic cloves, and honey in a small bowl.

6. Brush chicken with the glaze after the 20 minutes is over, flip the chicken so the breast side is now up, and brush the top with more glaze.

7. Set time to 25 more minutes and press Start/Pause. Glaze chicken every 5 minutes, or until all the glaze is used up.

8. Remove chicken when an instant-read meat thermometer inserted into the thickest part of the thigh registers 170°F. Transfer the chicken to a platter and tent with foil.

9. Place the chicken juices that were in the fryer basket into a saucepan. Simmer for 5 minutes. Place cornstarch in a small bowl and add 1 tablespoon of sauce. Whisk together and pour back into the saucepan. Continue to simmer until the sauce has thickened. Strain into a cup and discard the solids.

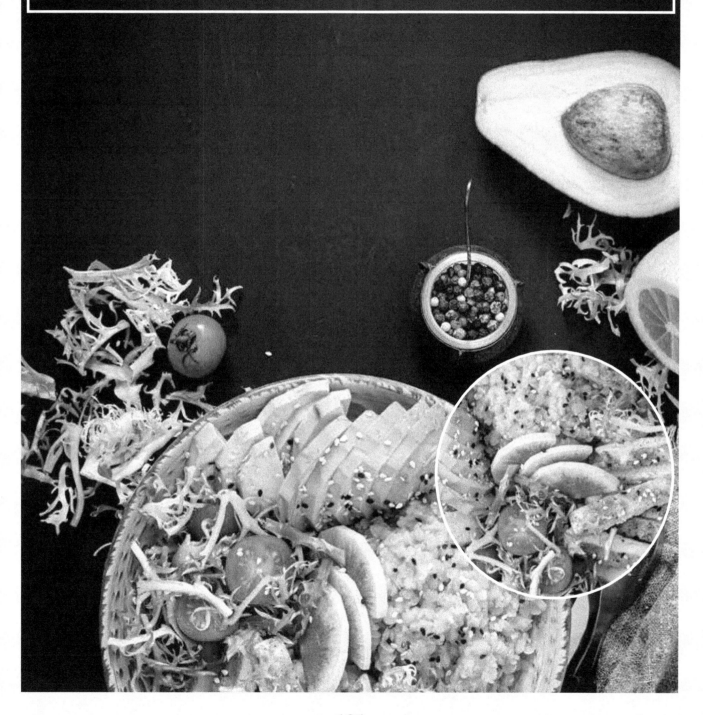

VEGETABLES RECIPES

Chestnut Stuffing

Cooking Time: 30 minutes   Servings: 5

INGREDIENTS

√ 2 ounces onion, minced
√ 2 ounces carrots, minced
√ 2 ounces celery, minced
√ 2 ounces white button mushrooms, minced
√ 1½ tablespoons unsalted butter or bacon fat
√ 12 ounces day-old bread, cubed
√ 4 fluid ounces chicken stock, hot
√ 1 egg, whisked
√ 2 tablespoons parsley
√ ½ teaspoon sage, chopped
√ 6 ounces shelled, peeled, roasted chestnuts, quartered
√ 1 teaspoon kosher salt
√ ½ teaspoon ground black pepper
√ 1 teaspoon ground nutmeg
√ ¼ teaspoon ground ginger
√ ¼ teaspoon ground mustard
√ Gravy, for serving (optional)

DIRECTIONS

1. Sauté the onions, carrots, celery, and mushrooms in the butter (or bacon fat) until tender, about 5 minutes.
2. Combine the bread, chicken stock, egg, and sauteed vegetables in a large bowl.
3. Add the parsley, sage, chestnuts, salt, pepper, nutmeg, ginger, and mustard and mix until fully combined.
4. Select the Preheat function on the Cosori Air Fryer, set temperature to 330°F, and press Start/Pause.
5. Line the preheated air fryer basket with foil, being careful not to touch the hot surfaces.
6. Transfer the stuffing into the lined air fryer basket.
7. Select the Bake function, adjust temperature to 330°F and time to 30 minutes, press Shake, then press Start/Pause.
8. Cover the top of the stuffing with foil halfway through cooking. The Shake Reminder will let you know when.
9. Let the stuffing cool for 5 minutes inside the air fryer basket, then transfer to a serving dish.
10. Scoop the stuffing out into a dish or flip the stuffing out onto a cutting board and cut into individual servings.
11. Serve alongside your Thanksgiving dinner with gravy, if desired.

Roasted Veggie Tacos

INGREDIENTS

√ 3 branches curly kale
√ 2 teaspoons olive oil, plus more as needed
√ 2 teaspoons salt, divided, plus more as needed
√ 1 small butternut squash
√ 1 teaspoon ground coriander, divided
√ ½ teaspoon cayenne pepper, divided
√ ½ teaspoon ground cinnamon, divided
√ ¼ teaspoon ground nutmeg, divided
√ 1 cup cauliflower florets
√ 1 tablespoon brown sugar
√ 8 corn tortillas, warmed
√ Red onion, thinly sliced, for serving
√ Queso fresco, for serving
√ For Serrano-Cilantro Avocado Crema:
√ 1 cup Mexican crema or sour cream
√ 2 teaspoons olive oil
√ 2 tablespoons cilantro, chopped
√ 1 lime, zested & juiced
√ 1 avocado
√ ½ serrano pepper, stem removed
√ A pinch of kosher salt

DIRECTIONS

1. Select the Preheat function on the Cosori Air Fryer, adjust temperature to 370°F, and press Start/Pause.
2. Wash and fully dry the kale leaves, then tear into 2-inch pieces.
3. Toss the torn kale with the olive oil and a pinch of salt, then gently massage the leaves to help the kale retain flavor.
4. Place the kale into the preheated air fryer baskets.
5. Set temperature to 370°F and time to 5 minutes, then press Start/Pause.
6. Remove kale when the leaves are crispy and sprinkle with kosher salt. Set aside.

7. Peel the butternut squash and cut in half lengthwise. Wear gloves to keep your hands from getting dried out.
8. Scoop the seeds out with a spoon and cut into ¼-inch batons. Set aside.
9. Combine 1 teaspoon salt, ½ teaspoon coriander, ¼ teaspoon cayenne pepper, ¼ teaspoon cinnamon, and ⅛ teaspoon ground nutmeg in a medium bowl with the cauliflower florets and mix well.
10. Add the butternut squash batons and the remaining salt, coriander, cayenne pepper, cinnamon, and nutmeg to the bowl and mix well.
11. Add 2 teaspoons of olive oil to the vegetable mixture and toss to coat.
12. Place the vegetable mixture into the preheated air fryer.
13. Set temperature to 400°F and time to 12 minutes, press Shake, then press Start/Pause.
14. Shake the veggies and add in the brown sugar halfway through cooking. The Shake Reminder will let you know when.
15. Blend together the Mexican crema or sour cream, olive oil, cilantro, lime juice and zest, avocado, and serrano pepper until smooth.
16. Remove the veggies when done.
17. Season the crema to taste with kosher salt and set aside.
18. Build the tacos by filling each tortilla with the roasted vegetables and topping with sliced red onion, the serrano-cilantro avocado crema, queso fresco, and the crispy kale, then serve.

Turkey Burgers with Asian Slaw

Cooking Time: 35 minutes   Servings: 4

INGREDIENTS

Asian Slaw
√ 2½ cups cabbage, shredded
√ ¼ small red onion, thinly sliced
√ ½ carrot, grated
√ 2 green onions, thinly sliced
√ 2 tablespoons cilantro, chopped
√ 2 tablespoons rice wine vinegar
√ 2 tablespoons soy sauce
√ 2 tablespoons brown sugar
√ 1 tablespoon sesame oil
√ Salt & pepper, to taste

Patty
√ 1 pound ground turkey (85/15)
√ 2 garlic cloves, minced
√ 1-inch piece ginger, grated
√ 2 green onions, chopped
√ 2 tablespoons hoisin
√ 1 tablespoon soy sauce
√ 2 teaspoons sambal oelek
√ ½ teaspoon salt
√ ¼ teaspoon black pepper
√ 1 cup panko breadcrumbs

DIRECTIONS

1. MIX together the cabbage, onion, carrots, green onions, and cilantro in a large bowl.

2. WHISK together the vinegar, soy sauce, brown sugar, sesame oil, mayonnaise, salt, and pepper in a small bowl.

3. TOSS the vegetables with the vinegar dressing and let the Asian slaw marinate for 30 minutes.

4. MIX all of the patty ingredients together in a large bowl until combined.

5. FORM the turkey mixture into 4 patties and set in the fridge to cool.

6. SELECT Preheat on the Cosori Air Fryer and press Start/Pause.

7. PLACE the turkey patties in the preheated air fryer.

8. COOK for 10 minutes at 400°F.

9. SERVE on buns with Asian slaw.

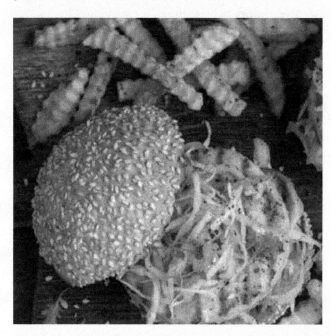

Teriyaki-Glazed Salmon

Cooking Time: 18 minutes   Servings: 2

INGREDIENTS

√ Teriyaki Sauce
√ ½ cup soy sauce
√ ¼ cup sugar
√ ¼ teaspoon grated ginger
√ 1 garlic clove, crushed
√ ¼ cup orange juice
√ Salmon
√ 2 salmon fillets (5 ounces)
√ 1 tablespoon vegetable oil
√ Salt & white pepper, to taste

DIRECTIONS

1. COMBINE all teriyaki sauce ingredients in a small sauce pot.

2. BRING the sauce to a boil, reduce by half, then let cool.

3. SELECT Preheat on the Cosori Air Fryer, adjust to 350°F, and press Start/Pause.

4. COAT the salmon with oil and season with salt and white pepper.

5. PLACE the salmon into the preheated air fryer, skin-side down. Select Seafood, adjust to 8 minutes, and press Start/Pause.

6. REMOVE the salmon from the air fryer when finished. Let rest for 5 minutes, then glaze with teriyaki sauce.

7. SERVE over a bed of white rice or with grilled vegetables.

Brussel Sprouts with Pancetta

Cooking Time: 13 minutes   Servings: 2-4

INGREDIENTS

√ 10 ounces brussel sprouts, halved
√ 2 strips pancetta, diced
√ 1 tablespoon olive oil
√ Salt & pepper, to taste
√ 1 tablespoon Parmesan cheese, freshly grated

DIRECTIONS

1. SELECT Preheat on the Cosori Air Fryer and press Start/Pause.

2. CUT the stems off of the brussel sprouts, then cut in half.

3. COMBINE brussel sprout halves, diced pancetta, olive oil, garlic powder, salt, and pepper in a bowl and mix together.

4. ADD mixture to the preheated air fryer.

5. SELECT Root Vegetables, adjust time to 8 minutes, then press Start/Pause. Make sure to shake the baskets halfway through cooking (the Shake Reminder function will let you know when!).

6. GRATE Parmesan cheese for garnish, then serve.

Roasted Butternut Squash

Cooking Time: 22 minutes   Servings: 2-4

INGREDIENTS
√ 1 butternut squash, peeled, seeded & cut into 1-inch cubes
√ 2 tablespoons olive oil, plus more for drizzling
√ 1½ teaspoons thyme leaves
√ 1 teaspoon salt
√ ½ teaspoon black pepper

DIRECTIONS
1. SELECT Preheat on the Cosori Air Fryer and press Start/Pause.
2. COAT the butternut squash cubes with olive oil and season with thyme, salt, and pepper.
3. ADD the seasoned squash to the preheated air fryer.
4. SELECT Root Vegetables and press Start/Pause. Make sure to shake the baskets halfway through cooking (the Shake Reminder function will let you know when!).
5. DRIZZLE with olive oil when done cooking and serve.

Roasted Corn

Cooking Time: 12 minutes   Servings: 2

INGREDIENTS
√ 1 ear of corn, husks & silks removed, cut in half
√ ¼ teaspoon salt
√ 1 tablespoon butter, melted

DIRECTIONS
1. SELECT Preheat on the Cosori Air Fryer, adjust to 400°F, and press Start/Pause.
2. BRUSH the melted butter all over the corn and season with salt.
3. PLACE the corn in the preheated air fryer.
4. SELECT Root Vegetables, adjust time to 10 minutes, and press Start/Pause.
5. FLIP the corn halfway through cooking (the Shake Reminder function will let you know when!).

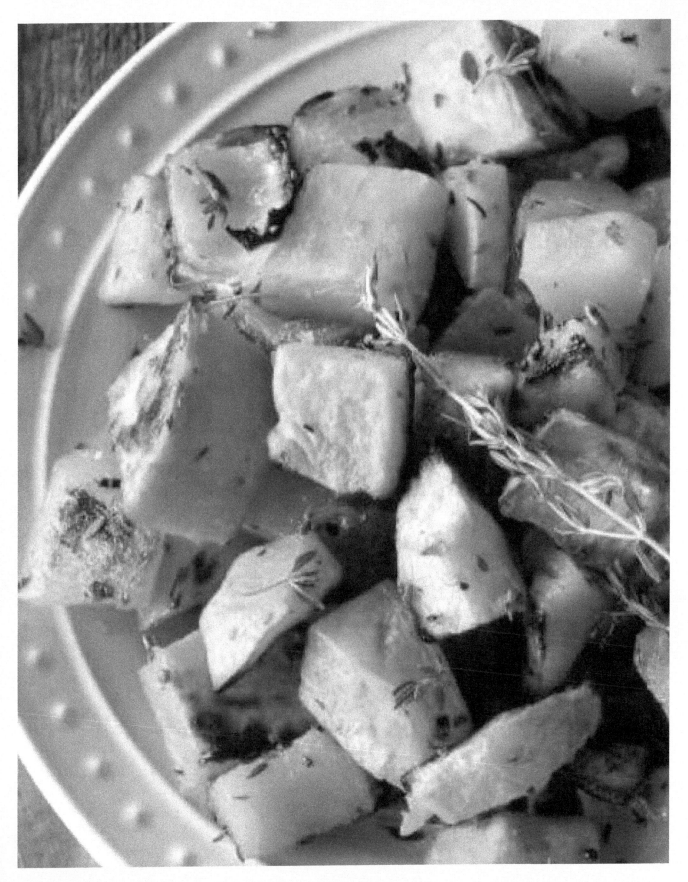

Roasted Turmeric Cauliflower

Cooking Time: 12 minutes   Servings: 2-3

INGREDIENTS
√ 10 ounces cauliflower florets
√ 2 teaspoons olive oil
√ 1 teaspoon turmeric powder
√ ½ teaspoon garlic powder
√ ½ teaspoon onion powder
√ ½ teaspoon salt
√ ¼ teaspoon black pepper

DIRECTIONS
1. SELECT Preheat on the Cosori Air Fryer, adjust to 300°F, and press Start/Pause.

2. PLACE the cauliflower florets into a bowl and drizzle with olive oil until all the cauliflower is well coated.
3. TOSS the cauliflower with the seasonings.
4. ADD the cauliflower into the preheated air fryer.
5. SELECT Vegetables, then press Start/Pause.

Beer Bratwurst with Onion and Peppers

Cooking Time: 42 minutes   Servings: 5

INGREDIENTS
√ 5 Bratwurst
√ 1 medium white onion, thinly sliced
√ 1 bell pepper, thinly sliced
√ 2 large garlic cloves, minced
√ 1 tablespoon butter
√ 1 tablespoon olive oil
√ 2 cups dark beer
√ ¼ cup brown sugar, packed
√ 2 tablespoons apple cider vinegar
√ 1 teaspoon black pepper
√ 4 sliced sandwich rolls, toasted
√ Sauerkraut, for topping (optional)
√ Spicy brown mustard, for topping (optional)
√ Cosori 7-inch Cake Pan Accessory

DIRECTIONS
1. Select the Preheat function on the Cosori Air Fryer, and press Start/Pause.
2. Place the butter, olive oil, garlic, sliced onion and bell peppers in the Cosori cake pan accessory.
3. Insert pan into the preheated air fryer basket.

Select the Root Vegetables function on the Cosori Air Fryer, and press Start/Pause. Stir the mixture halfway through cooking.
4. Remove pan and add the beer, brown sugar, apple cider vinegar, black pepper, and stir together. Submerge the bratwurst into the liquid mixture. Cover the pan with foil and insert back into the air fryer.
5. Set the temperature to 400°F, time to 15 minutes, and press Start/Pause. Remove foil and cook for an additional 5 minutes.
6. Remove pan from the fryer basket. Add only the bratwurst back into the fryer basket. Reserve the onions and peppers for serving and discard the liquid.
7. Set the temperature to 400°F, time to 5 minutes, and press Start/Pause. Remove when the Bratwurst are golden brown.
8. Serve Bratwurst in toasted sandwich rolls with onions and peppers, spicy brown mustard, and sauerkraut.

Roasted Cauliflower

Cooking Time: 12 minutes   Servings: 2-3

INGREDIENTS

√ 10 ounces cauliflower florets
√ ½ teaspoon salt
√ 2 teaspoons olive oil
√ ¼ teaspoon black pepper

DIRECTIONS

1. SELECT Preheat on the Cosori Air Fryer, adjust to 300°F, and press Start/Pause.
2. PLACE the cauliflower florets into a bowl, drizzle with olive oil, and season with salt and pepper, tossing to coat the florets evenly.
3. ADD the cauliflower into the preheated air fryer.
4. SELECT Vegetables, then press Start/Pause.

Honey Soy Carrots

Cooking Time: 17 minutes   Servings: 4

INGREDIENTS

√ 1 pound young carrots (6-inch), rinsed, scrubbed clean & patted dry
√ 1 teaspoon honey
√ 1 tablespoon olive oil
√ 1 teaspoon soy sauce
√ Salt & pepper, to taste

DIRECTIONS

1. SELECT Preheat on the Cosori Air Fryer and press Start/Pause.
2. COAT the carrots in olive oil and toss in the honey and soy sauce
3. PLACE the carrots in the preheated air fryer.
4. SELECT Root Vegetables and press Start/Pause.
Make sure to shake the baskets halfway through cooking (the Shake Reminder function will let you know when!).
5. SEASON with salt and pepper when done cooking.

129

Roasted Garlic Broccoli

Cooking Time: 13 minutes   Servings: 3

INGREDIENTS

√ 1 large head broccoli, cut into florets
√ 1 teaspoon garlic powder
√ ¼ teaspoon black pepper
√ 1 tablespoon olive oil
√ ½ teaspoon salt

DIRECTIONS

1. SELECT Preheat on the Cosori Air Fryer, adjust to 300°F, and press Start/Pause.

2. DRIZZLE the broccoli with olive oil and toss together until evenly coated.

3. TOSS the broccoli with the seasonings.

4. ADD the broccoli to the preheated air fryer.

5. SELECT Vegetables and press Start/Pause.

Roasted Rainbow Carrots

Cooking Time: 15 minutes   Servings: 2-4

INGREDIENTS

√ 1 pound heirloom rainbow carrots, peeled & washed
√ 2 teaspoons olive oil
√ 2 sprigs fresh thyme, stripped
√ 1 tablespoon fresh tarragon leaves, chopped
√ ½ teaspoon kosher salt
√ ¼ teaspoon freshly ground black pepper

DIRECTIONS

1. Pat the peeled and washed carrots dry with a paper towel. Set aside.

2. Select the Preheat function on the Cosori Air Fryer, set temperature to 400°F, then press Start/Pause.

3. Toss carrots with olive oil, thyme, tarragon, salt, and pepper in a bowl.

4. Place carrots into the preheated air fryer.

5. Select the Root Vegetables function, set time to 10 minutes, then press Start/Pause. The Shake Reminder will prompt you to shake the baskets halfway through cooking.

6. Remove when done and serve hot.

Honey-Roasted Carrots

Cooking Time: 17 minutes   Servings: 2-4

INGREDIENTS
√ 1 pound heirloom rainbow carrots, peeled & washed
√ 1 tablespoon olive oil
√ 2 tablespoons honey
√ 2 sprigs fresh thyme
√ Salt & pepper, to taste

DIRECTIONS
1. PAT DRY the carrots with a paper towel. Set aside.
2. SELECT Preheat on the Cosori Air Fryer and press Start/Pause.
3. TOSS the carrots in a bowl with olive oil, honey, thyme, salt, and pepper.
4. ADD the carrots to the preheated air fryer.
5. SELECT Root Vegetables and press Start/Pause. Make sure to shake the baskets halfway through cooking (the Shake Reminder function will let you know when!).
6. SERVE hot.

Roasted Butternut Squash with Sweetcorn Salsa

Cooking Time: 22 minutes   Servings: 4-6

INGREDIENTS
√ 1 butternut squash, peeled, halved lengthwise, & de-seeded
√ 2 tablespoons olive oil
√ ½ teaspoon kosher salt
√ ¼ teaspoon ground paprika
√ ¼ teaspoon ground cumin
√ 2 tablespoons fresh cilantro, chopped
√ Pumpkin Seeds, toasted, for garnish
√ A pinch of black pepper
√ A pinch of ground cinnamon
√ A pinch of cayenne pepper
√ 1 cup corn kernels, cooked
√ 1 lime, juiced
√ Salt & pepper, to taste
√ Cotija cheese, crumbled, for garnish

DIRECTIONS
1. Cut the butternut squash into ½-inch-thick slices.
2. Select the Preheat function on the Cosori Air Fryer, set temperature to 400°F, then press Start/Pause.
3. Toss the sliced squash with olive oil, salt, paprika, cumin, black pepper, cinnamon, and cayenne pepper. Set aside.
4. Place the seasoned squash into the preheated air fryer.
5. Select the Root Vegetables function, then press Start/Pause. The Shake Reminder will prompt you to shake the baskets halfway through cooking.
6. Mix together cooked corn kernels, lime juice, and chopped cilantro to make sweetcorn salsa.
7. Season the salsa with salt and pepper to taste. Set aside.
8. Garnish the roasted squash with corn salsa, Cotija cheese, and toasted pumpkin seeds, then serve.

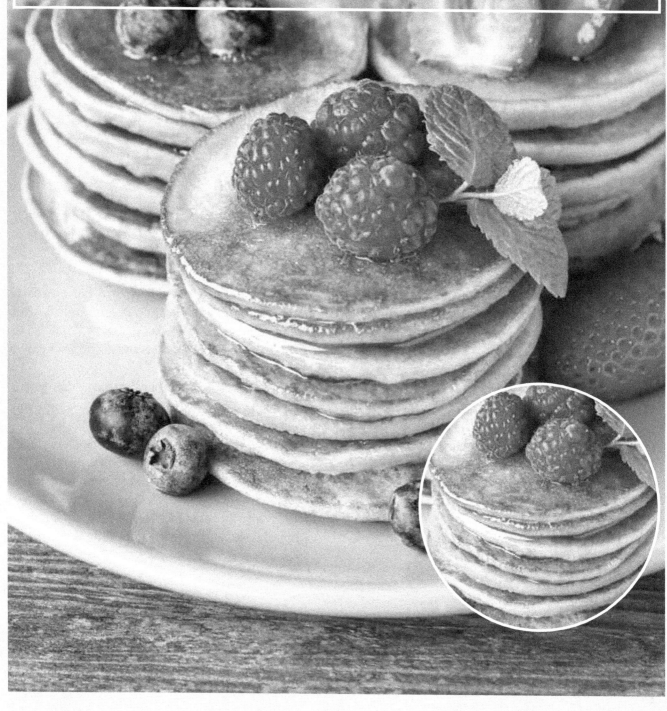

DESSERT RECIPES

Guinness Extra Stout Double Chocolate Brownies

INGREDIENTS

√ 1 cup all-purpose flour, plus more for dusting

√ ¾ cup unsweetened cocoa powder

√ 1 teaspoon kosher salt

√ 6 tablespoons unsalted butter, cubed

√ 8 ounces dark chocolate chips (70% cocoa), chopped

√ ¾ cup white chocolate chips

√ 4 large eggs

√ ¾ cup granulated white sugar

√ 10 ounces Guinness® Extra Stout Beer, flat and room-temperature

√ ½ cup mini semi-sweet chocolate chips

√ Items Needed:

√ 1 square cake pan (8 x 8 inches)

√ Parchment paper

√ Electric hand mixer

DIRECTIONS

1. Butter the sides of the cake pan and dust with flour.

2. Cut out a square piece of parchment paper fitted to the bottom of the pan and place inside.

3. Combine the flour, cocoa powder, and salt in a medium bowl and set aside.

4. Melt the butter, dark chocolate chips, and white chocolate chips in a double-boiler over low heat. Stir constantly until silky smooth, then remove from heat.

5. Whisk the eggs and sugar together using an electric hand mixer on high speed until pale and fluffy, about 3 minutes.

6. Temper the eggs by whisking in 1/3 of the chocolate mixture. Once fully combined, whisk in the rest of the chocolate.

7. Fold in the flour mixture to the chocolate mixture. Once combined, slowly whisk in the flat, room-temperature beer.

8. Pour the batter into the prepared cake pan and top with mini semi-sweet chocolate chips.

9. Place only the cooking pot into the base of the Cosori Smart Indoor Grill.

10. Select the Bake function, adjust temperature to 375°F and time to 20 minutes, then press Start/Pause to preheat.

11. Place the brownie pan into the preheated cooking pot, then close the lid.

12. Remove the brownies when done, or until a skewer or cake tester comes out clean, then let the brownies cool to room temperature before slicing.

13. Serve warm.

Chocolate Lava Cakes

INGREDIENTS

√ 3 tablespoons unsalted butter, room temperature, plus more for ramekins

√ 3 tablespoons granulated sugar, plus more for ramekins

√ 3 ounces bittersweet chocolate, chopped

√ 1 large whole egg, plus 1 large egg yolk

√ ⅛ teaspoon kosher salt

√ ½ teaspoon vanilla extract

√ 2 tablespoons all-purpose flour

√ Confectioner's sugar, for serving

√ Items Needed:

√ 2 ramekins (6 ounces each)

√ Electric hand mixer

√ Sieve

DIRECTIONS

1. Grease each ramekin with butter, then dust lightly with sugar. Tap out the extra sugar and set aside.

2. Place chocolate and butter in a heatproof bowl.

3. Melt the chocolate butter mixture in a double boiler (over simmering water), then remove from heat.

4. Select the Preheat function on the Cosori Smart Air Fryer, adjust temperature to 360°F, then press Start/Pause.

5. Place the whole egg, egg yolk, sugar, and salt in a medium bowl. Beat at high speed using an electric hand mixer until thickened and pale in color.

6. Add the vanilla extract, chocolate butter mixture, and flour to the bowl and whisk until smooth.

7. Spoon batter into the prepared ramekins.

8. Place the ramekins into the preheated air fryer.

9. Set temperature to 360°F and time to 9 minutes, then press Start/Pause.

10. Remove lava cakes when done, or firm with a soft center. Let cool in the ramekins for 1 minute before carefully inverting onto a plate.

11. Dust with confectioners' sugar using a sieve and serve.

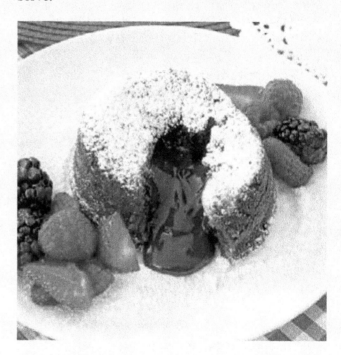

Cranberry Apple Crisp

Cooking Time: 30 minutes   Servings: 6-8

INGREDIENTS
Filling:
√ 1½ cups fresh cranberries
√ 2 Granny Smith apples, cut into 1-inch cubes
√ 2 Gala apples (Fuji or Pink Lady), cut into 1-inch cubes
√ ¼ cup maple syrup
√ 3 tablespoons brown sugar
√ 1 tablespoon cane sugar
√ ½ teaspoon cinnamon
√ ½ teaspoon allspice
√ ½ teaspoon lemon juice
√ 2 tablespoons cornstarch
√ ¼ teaspoon salt
√ Oil spray

Topping:
√ 1½ cups rolled oats
√ 1/3 cup brown sugar
√ 4 tablespoons flour
√ 4 tablespoons coconut oil, melted
√ ¼ teaspoon cinnamon
√ A pinch of salt
√ Non-dairy or low-calorie ice cream, for serving (optional)

DIRECTIONS
1. Combine all the ingredients for the filling except the oil spray in a large bowl and set aside.
2. Mix the ingredients for the toppings thoroughly in a separate medium bowl.
3. Coat the Cosori Smart Air Fryer basket with oil spray.
4. Pour the filling mixture directly into the air fryer basket, without the crisper plate. Spread the mixture evenly.
5. Sprinkle the topping across the top of the filling mixture.
6. Select the Bake function, adjust temperature to 325°F and time to 30 minutes, then press Start/Pause.
7. Remove the cranberry apple crisp when done and serve warm with your choice of ice cream.

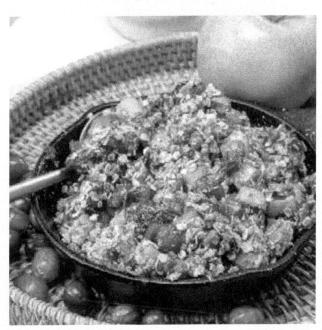

Salted Caramel Snickerdoodle Skillet Cookie

Cooking Time: 23 minutes   Servings: 4

INGREDIENTS

√ 2¾ cups all-purpose flour
√ 2 teaspoons cream of tartar
√ 1 teaspoon baking soda
√ ½ teaspoon kosher salt
√ 1 teaspoon ground cinnamon, plus more for serving
√ 1½ cups granulated sugar
√ 4 ounces unsalted butter, room temperature
√ 1 teaspoon vanilla extract
√ 2 large eggs
√ ½ cup salted caramel, plus more for serving
√ Vanilla ice cream, for serving

ITEMS NEEDED:

√ Stand mixer fitted with paddle attachment
√ Cast iron skillet (6-inch diameter) or cake pan

DIRECTIONS

1. Whisk the flour, cream of tartar, baking soda, salt, and cinnamon together in a medium bowl.

2. Cream the sugar and butter together in a stand mixer fitted with the paddle attachment, then add the vanilla extract.

3. Add the eggs, one at a time, until fully combined, scraping down the sides of the bowl as needed with a rubber spatula.

4. Add the dry ingredients to the stand mixer and beat on low just until combined. Add the salted caramel and stir to swirl it into the dough, but do not mix it in completely.

5. Fill the skillet or cake pan 2/3 full with dough. Reserve the remaining dough in the refrigerator for a second batch of cookies later.

6. Place the cooking pot into the base of the Cosori Indoor Grill, followed by the basket.

7. Select the Bake function, adjust temperature to 320°F and time to 20 minutes, then press Start/Pause to preheat.

8. Place the skillet or cake pan into the preheated basket, then close the lid.

9. Select the Broil function, adjust time 3 minutes, then press Start/Pause.

10. Remove the skillet or cake pan when done and let cool slightly.

11. Serve the cookie in slices, drizzled with salted caramel sauce, sprinkled with cinnamon, and a scoop of vanilla ice cream on top.

Apple Tart

INGREDIENTS

√ 1 premade 8-inch pie crust, room temperature
√ 250 grams gala and granny smith apples (about 4 small apples)
√ 1 lemon, juiced
√ 2 teaspoons kosher salt
√ Items Needed:
√ Cosori baking sheet accessory
√ Kitchen scale
√ 3 tablespoons apricot preserves
√ 3 tablespoons turbinado sugar
√ 4 tablespoons frozen unsalted butter, cut into small cubes

DIRECTIONS

1. Select the Preheat function on the Cosori Smart Air Fryer Toaster Oven, adjust temperature to 400°F, and press Start/Pause.

2. Poke holes across the bottom of the pie crust using a fork. This will prevent the pie crust from puffing up and changing shape.

3. Core the apples and slice them into ¼-inch-thick slices.

4. Combine the lemon juice, salt, and apple slices in a large bowl. Add enough water to cover the apples.

5. Place the pie crust onto the baking sheet, then insert the baking sheet at mid position in the preheated oven.

6. Select the Bake function, adjust temperature to 400°F and time to 5 minutes, then press Start/Pause.

7. Remove the pie crust when done, and set aside to cool for 5 minutes.

8. Mix the apricot preserves with 1 tablespoon of water in a small bowl. Microwave for 30 seconds, then stir well.

9. Drain the apple slices from the water and shake off excess water.

10. Brush a layer of loosened apricot preserves across the entire surface of the cooled pie crust.

11. Layer the apple slices in concentric circles inside the crust to form a rose-like pattern, alternating apple colors if desired. Using the same process, create a second layer to fill the crust to the top.

Note: There should be a hole in the center of both layers where the ring of apples becomes too tight to continue making circles.

12. Create a "rose bud" in the center by laying down 2 apple slices vertically into the hole, each slice mirroring the other to create a circle. Afterwards, stand up 3 apple slices to lean against each other horizontally over the apple circle.

13. Brush the top of the apples with the loosened apricot preserves, then sprinkle with turbinado sugar and cubed butter.

14. Place the tart onto the baking sheet, then insert the baking sheet at mid position into the preheated oven.

15. Select the Bake function, adjust temperature to 375°F and time to 30 minutes, press Shake, then press Start/Pause.

16. Tent the top with aluminum foil halfway through cooking. The Shake Reminder will let you know when.

17. Remove when done and let cool completely before slicing and serving.

Sweet Potato Cornbread

Cooking Time: 35 minutes   Servings: 8

INGREDIENTS

√ ¾ cup yellow cornmeal
√ ½ cup all-purpose flour
√ ¼ cup white granulated sugar
√ 1½ teaspoons baking powder
√ ½ teaspoon kosher salt
√ ¼ teaspoon cinnamon
√ ¼ teaspoon nutmeg
√ 8 ounces sweet potato, mashed
√ Items Needed:
√ 8-inch cake pan
√ 1 large egg
√ 1/3 cup milk
√ ¼ cup sour cream
√ 1 can sweet corn, drained
√ 1 tablespoon vegetable oil
√ 1 tablespoon unsalted butter, for pan
√ 1 tablespoon cornmeal, for dusting the pan
√ Butter, warmed, for serving (optional)

DIRECTIONS

1. Combine the cornmeal, flour, sugar, baking powder, salt, cinnamon, and nutmeg in a medium bowl, then set aside.

2. Whisk the sweet potato, egg, milk, sour cream, sweet corn and vegetable oil together in a separate large bowl until smooth.

3. Add the dry mixture to the wet mixture and mix just until combined.

4. Grease an 8-inch cake pan with butter and dust with cornmeal. Tap the pan to spread the cornmeal evenly across the bottom.

5. Cover the cake pan with aluminum foil.

6. Select the Preheat function on the Cosori Smart Air Fryer Toaster Oven, adjust temperature to 400°F, and press Start/Pause.

7. Insert the cake pan at mid position in the preheated oven.

8. Select the Bake function, adjust temperature to 400°F and time to 35 minutes, press Shake, then press Start/Pause.

9. Remove the aluminum foil cover halfway through cooking. The Shake Reminder will let you know when.

10. Remove the cornbread when done and let cool for 5 minutes, then remove the cornbread from the pan and set on a wire rack to cool completely.

11. Slice into 9 pieces and serve at room temperature or warmed with butter, if desired.

Cherry Hand Pies

Cooking Time: 8 minutes   Servings: 14

INGREDIENTS
Cherry Hand Pie:
√ 12 ounces frozen or fresh cherries, pitted
√ 1 tablespoon lemon juice
√ ¼ cup granulated sugar
√ A pinch of kosher salt
√ 1 tablespoon cornstarch
√ ½ teaspoon almond extract
√ 2 sheets frozen puff pastry, thawed
√ 1 egg, beaten
Glaze:
√ 1 cup powdered sugar
√ 1 tablespoon whole milk
√ ½ teaspoon vanilla extract
√ Items Needed:
√ Rolling pin
√ 3-inch round cutter
√ Baking sheet
√ Wax paper

DIRECTIONS
1. Combine the cherries, lemon juice, sugar, and salt in a saucepan over medium-high heat. Bring mixture to a boil, then reduce to a simmer for 5 minutes.
2. Smash some of the cherries lightly with a fork.
3. Place the cornstarch in a small bowl. Add 3 tablespoons of the cherry liquid and stir until no clumps remain.
4. Pour the cornstarch mixture into the saucepan and stir. When the mixture thickens, remove from heat, stir in the almond extract, and refrigerate until slightly chilled.
5. Roll out each puff pastry sheet on a floured surface into a 9 x 12-inch rectangle. Using a 3-inch round cutter, cut out circles in the puff pastry.
6. Place the circles onto a baking sheet lined with wax paper.
7. Spoon about 2 teaspoons of cherry filling onto half of the puff pastry circles. Brush the edges with some of the beaten egg and place the remaining puff pastry circles on top to enclose.
8. Press the edges with a fork to seal. Refrigerate for 20 minutes.
9. Select the Preheat function on the Cosori Air Fryer, adjust temperature to 350°F, and press Start/Pause.
10. Cut a 1-inch vent in the top of each pastry. Brush the tops with more of the beaten egg.
11. Place the cherry hand pies into the preheated fryer baskets.
12. Set time to 8 minutes, then press Start/Pause.
13. Remove when golden and puffed. Transfer to a wire rack immediately and allow to cool completely.
14. Whisk the glaze ingredients together in a small bowl until smooth, then glaze the cooled cherry hand pies.
15. Serve the pies when the glaze is set.

Spooky Ghost Puffs

Cooking Time: 12 minutes   Servings: 9

INGREDIENTS

Puff:

√ 2 ½ ounces whole milk

√ 2 ½ ounces water

√ 1/8 teaspoon kosher salt

√ 2.5 ounces unsalted butter

√ 76 grams bread flour

√ 150 grams whisked eggs

√ White Chocolate Ganache:

√ 1 ½ cups white chocolate chips

√ ½ cup heavy whipping cream

√ Raspberry

Mascarpone Filling:

√ 1 cup mascarpone, room temperature

√ 1 cup heavy cream

√ 2 tablespoons powdered sugar

√ 1 teaspoon vanilla extract

√ 1/3 cup raspberry preserves

DIRECTIONS

1. Bring the milk, water, salt, and butter to boil over medium heat, stirring constantly. When the butter melts, add the flour in all at once and stir vigorously until fully combined. When the mixture forms a mass and pulls away from the sides of the pan, remove from heat and place into the stand mixer bowl.

2. Use the paddle attachment and beat on medium speed. Add the whisked eggs in 3 different additions, ensuring that the eggs fully incorporate into the dough before adding the next addition.

3. When the dough develops a pearl like sheen and is firm enough to hold its shape when piped, it's ready.

4. Place the dough into a large piping bag and snip about 1-inch off the tip.

5. Pipe onto parchment paper and set aside.

6. Select the Preheat function on the Cosori Air Fryer, adjust temperature to 350°F, and press Start/Pause.

7. Place the piped puffs into the preheated air fryer basket.

8. Set temperature to 350°F, time to 12 minutes, enable the Shake function and press Start/Pause. Do not open the air fryer during the cooking process or the puffs will deflate. Once the puffs are done, leave them in the air fryer for 2 minutes after the timer goes off.

9. Remove from the air fryer and let cool on a wire rack.

10. Make the raspberry mascarpone filling: Beat mascarpone with the paddle attachment using an electric mixer on low speed. Remove the whipped mascarpone and set aside. Add the heavy cream, vanilla, and powdered sugar into the stand mixer bowl. Beat on medium until the mixture forms medium peaks then remove from mixer and fold in the mascarpone. Lastly add the raspberry jam and gently fold until combined. Place into a large piping bag fitted with a #9 star tip. Keep refrigerated until ready to use.

11. Make the white chocolate ganache: Bring the heavy whipping cream just to a simmer in a small saucepan over medium heat. Place white chocolate chips in a bowl and pour the hot cream over. Let sit for 5 minutes. Whisk gently to combine.

12. Pipe the raspberry mascarpone into the puffs by inserting it from the bottom of the puff.

13. Dip the tops into the white chocolate ganache and decorate with candy eyes.

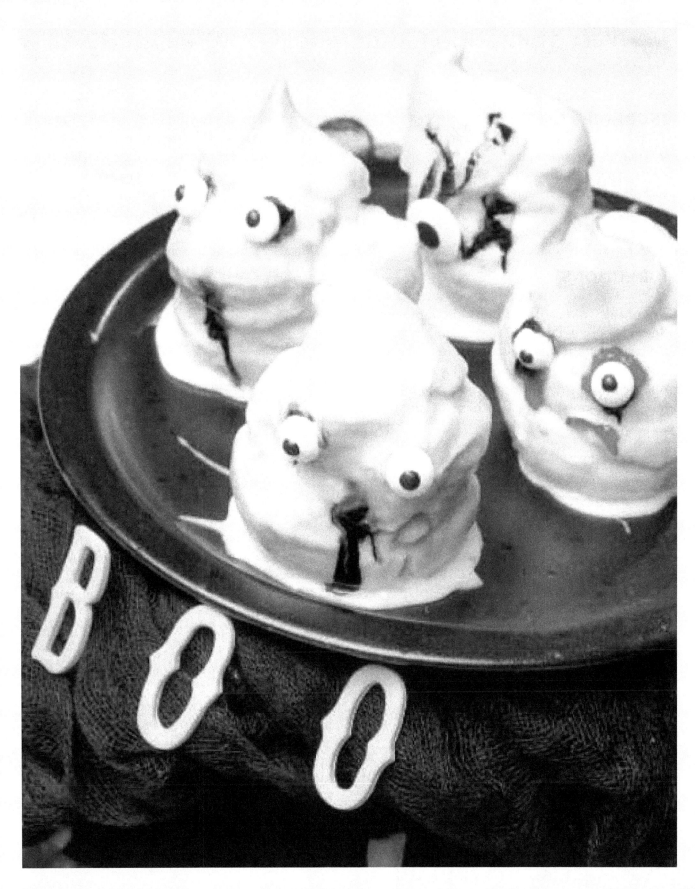

Bloody Witch Finger Cookies

Cooking Time: 7 minutes   Servings: 30

INGREDIENTS
√ 16 ounce package pre-made sugar cookie dough
√ 1 cup all-purpose flour
√ 3 teaspoons water
√ 5 Oreo cookies, ground up into crumbs in a food processor
√ ½ cup raspberry jam
√ ½ cup sliced almonds

DIRECTIONS
1. Place sugar cookie dough, flour, water, and ¼ cup of the Oreo cookie crumbs in a large bowl. Knead with your hands or in a stand mixer until all the ingredients are incorporated into the dough.
2. Take 1 ½ tablespoons of dough at a time and roll the dough between your palms into a 5-inch longer finger about ¼-inch thick. Firmly press a sliced almond into the end of each finger to make fingernails. Make several horizontal cuts in the center of each finger to make knuckles. Place fingers on a wax paper lined baking sheet.
3. Select the Preheat function on the Cosori Air Fryer, adjust temperature to 320°F, and press Start/Pause.
4. Place fingers into the preheated air fryer basket. You will need to work in batches.
5. Set the temperature to 320°F, time to 7 minutes, and press Start/Pause.
6. Remove fingers when lightly golden and place on a wire rack to cool completely.
7. Heat the raspberry jam in a saucepan or microwave until gently warmed through.
8. Dip the end of each finger into the raspberry jam and place onto a serving platter.

Chocolate Cake

Cooking Time: 65 minutes   Servings: 6

INGREDIENTS
Cake
√ 1 cup flour
√ 1/3 cup cocoa powder
√ ½ teaspoon baking soda
√ 1 teaspoon baking powder
√ 3 eggs, beaten
√ 2/3 cup sugar
√ ½ cup butter, softened
√ ½ cup sour cream
√ 1 teaspoon vanilla extract
√ Cooking spray
Frosting
√ 1 cup icing powdered sugar, plus more for dusting
√ 2 tablespoons cocoa powder
√ 4 tablespoons heavy cream

DIRECTIONS
1. Combine flour, cocoa powder, baking soda, and baking powder and mix.
2. Mix eggs, sugar, butter, sour cream, and vanilla extract in a separate bowl.
3. Fold the wet ingredients into the dry ingredients until well combined.
4. Select Preheat on the Cosori Air Fryer, adjust to 300°F, and press Start/Pause.
5. Spray the Cosori Cake Tin liberally with nonstick cooking spray.
6. Pour the cake batter into the cake tin and place into the preheated air fryer baskets.
7. Select Desserts, adjust time to 40 minutes, and press Start/Pause.
8. Remove cake tin from the air fryer when done cooking and allow to rest for 15 minutes.
9. Combine frosting ingredients and mix until well combined. Then, spread frosting onto the cake.
10. Dust more powdered sugar on top and serve.

Vegan Chocolate Chip Cookies

Cooking Time: 10 minutes   Servings: 24

INGREDIENTS

√ ¼ cup + 1 tablespoon refined coconut oil, melted
√ 3 tablespoons smooth almond butter
√ ¼ cup sugar (vegan)
√ ¼ cup + 2 tablespoons dark brown sugar, packed (vegan)
√ 2 tablespoons water
√ 2 tablespoons almond milk
√ 1 teaspoon vanilla extract
√ 1 ¼ cups all-purpose flour
√ ½ teaspoon baking soda
√ ½ teaspoon baking powder
√ ½ teaspoon salt
√ ½ cup dark chocolate chips (vegan)
√ ½ cup semi sweet chocolate chips (vegan)
√ Flakey sea salt for topping (optional)

DIRECTIONS

1. Combine melted coconut oil, almond butter, sugar, brown sugar, water, almond milk, and vanilla in a large mixing bowl. Whisk to combine.
2. Add flour, baking soda, baking powder, and salt. Fold to combine.
3. Fold in chocolate chips.
4. Refrigerate dough for 1 hour.
5. Scoop dough into 1 ½ inch balls.
6. Select Preheat on the Cosori air fryer, change temperature to 320°F, and press Start/Pause.
7. Place cookie balls in the fryer basket lined with parchment paper. Lightly flatten the cookies with the palm of your hand. Sprinkle with flakey sea salt (optional).
8. Set the temperature to 320°F, time to 7 minutes, and press Start/Pause.
9. Remove cookies when set and golden on top.
10. Allow cookies to cool for 5 minutes before enjoying.

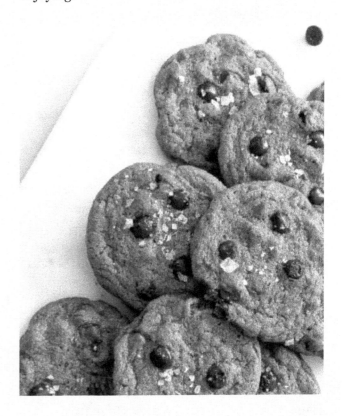

Fudgy Flourless Brownies

INGREDIENTS

√ 1 stick unsalted butter
√ 3 large eggs
√ ½ cup granulated sugar
√ ½ cup dark brown sugar, packed
√ 1 cup chocolate chips
√ 2 tablespoons cocoa powder
√ 2 teaspoons vanilla extract
√ 1 tablespoon brewed espresso
√ 1 tablespoon hot water
√ 1 cup almond flour
√ ½ teaspoon kosher salt

DIRECTIONS

1. Beat together the sugars and eggs using an electric mixer on high speed for 2 minutes, or until the mixture becomes pale in color and has slightly thickened.

2. Melt the butter in a small saucepan over medium-low heat. Place the chocolate chips in a bowl and pour the hot melted butter over the chocolate chips. Stir until the chocolate is melted.

3. Add the cocoa powder, vanilla extract, espresso, and hot water in a separate bowl. Stir together.

4. Add the melted chocolate mixture and cocoa powder mixture to the bowl with the egg and sugar mixture. Beat on medium speed until incorporated. Add the almond flour and salt and beat on low speed until combined.

5. Select Preheat on the Cosori Air Fryer, adjust temperature to 320°F, and press Start/Pause.

6. Grease a 7-inch round or square baking pan.

Pour the brownie batter in the baking pan. Insert the baking pan into the fryer basket and place in the air fryer.

7. Set temperature to 320°F, time to 50 minutes, and press Start/Pause.

8. Remove when a toothpick inserted into the middle comes out mostly clean with a few crumbs.

9. Allow the brownies to cool at room temperature for 30 minutes before slicing. Store brownies in the refrigerator to get clean slices.

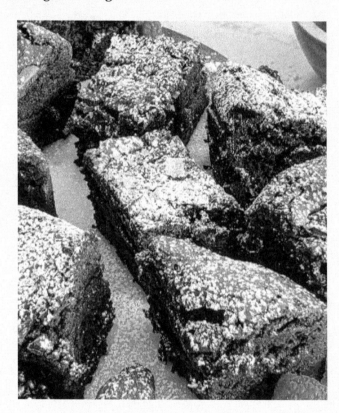

144

Swedish Almond Cranberry Cake

Cooking Time: 170 minutes   Servings: 6

INGREDIENTS

Cake
√ 1/3 cup plain yogurt, plus 1 tablespoon
√ ¾ cup granulated sugar
√ 2 large eggs
√ ¾ cup all purpose flour, sifted
√ 1/3 cup almond flour, plus 1 tablespoon
√ 1½ teaspoons baking powder, sifted
√ ½ teaspoon salt
√ ½ teaspoon almond extract
√ 1 teaspoon vanilla extract
√ 1/3 cup canola oil, plus 1 tablespoon
√ 1/3 cup dried cranberries

Glaze
√ ½ teaspoon finely grated orange zest
√ ¾ tablespoon fresh orange juice
√ ½ cup powdered sugar
√ ¼ teaspoon vanilla extract
√ ¼ teaspoon almond extract
√ 1/3 cups slivered almonds, toasted

DIRECTIONS

1. Combine the orange zest, orange juice, powdered sugar, vanilla extract, and almond extract in a small microwaveable bowl for the glaze and whisk until smooth. Set aside.

2. Whisk together yogurt, sugar, and eggs until smooth.

3. Add the all-purpose flour, almond flour, baking powder, salt and extracts. Stir to combine.

4. Add the oil and whisk until smooth.

5. Sprinkle the cranberries lightly with flour and fold into the cake batter.

6. Spray the Cosori cake pan accessory with cooking spray and pour the batter into the cake pan accessory.

7. Select the Preheat function on the Cosori Air Fryer, adjust to 300°F, and press Start/Pause.

8. Place the cake into the preheated air fryer basket.

9. Select the Bake function and press Start/Pause.

10. Cool cake the cake on a wire rack when done cooking for 10 minutes.

11. Turn the cake onto the wire rack and set the cake top side up.

12. Brush the cake with the all glaze while it is still warm allowing it to drip off to the sides.

13. Evenly scatter the toasted almonds on the top of the cake while it is still wet and gently press down.

14. Allow the cake to cool completely for 2 hours.

15. Sprinkle powdered sugar on top and serve.

Lemon & Thyme Yogurt Cake

Cooking Time: 120 minutes   Servings: 8

INGREDIENTS

Cake
√ ½ cup plain yogurt
√ 1 cup granulated sugar
√ 3 large eggs
√ 1½ cups all-purpose flour
√ 2 teaspoons baking powder
√ ½ teaspoon kosher salt
√ 1 lemon, zested
√ 6 springs of fresh thyme leaves
√ ½ cup olive oil
√ Cooking spray

Glaze
√ ¼ cup fresh lemon juice
√ ¾ cup of powdered sugar

DIRECTIONS

1. Whisk together plain yogurt, sugar, and eggs in a large bowl until well combined.

2. Sift in the flour and baking powder into the wet batter.

3. Whisk in the kosher salt, lemon zest, thyme leaves, and olive oil until smooth. Set aside.

4. Spray the cake pan accessory lightly with coking spray and cover the bottom with a round piece of parchemnt paper.

5. Select the Preheat function on the Cosori Air Fryer, adjust to 300F, and press Start/Pause.

6. Pour the batter into the Cosori cake pan accessory and place into the preheated air fryer basket.

7. Bake for 50 minutes or until the cake feels springy to the touch and a toothpick isnerted into the center comes out clean.

8. cool cake on a wire rack for 10 minutes; then turn it out of the pan onto the rack.

9. Combine the lemon juice and powdered sugar in a microwaveable safe small bowl.

10. Microwave the glaze in for 30 seconds, then mix well until smooth.

11. Brush the glaze all over the cake until all of the glaze is gone. (Some of it will drip off, but most of it will soak in.) Allow the cake to cool, about 1 hour.

12. Sprinkle with powdered sugar if desired and serve.

Caramel Swirl Brownies

Cooking Time: 160 minutes   Servings: 12

INGREDIENTS

√ 2/3 cup butter, melted
√ 1 cup granulated sugar
√ ½ teaspoon vanilla extract
√ 3 large eggs
√ ¾ cups all-purpose flour
√ 1/3 teaspoon baking powder
√ ½ cup extra dark cocoa powder
√ ¼ teaspoon instant espresso
√ 1/3 teaspoon kosher salt
√ 6 tablespoons caramel sauce

DIRECTIONS

1. Whisk together melted butter, granulated sugar, vanilla extract, and eggs in a large bowl until smooth. Set aside.

2. Whisk the flour, baking powder, cocoa powder, instant espresso, and salt until well combined.

3. Fold the dry ingredients into the wet ingredients until the flour is fully incorporated.

4. Mix the brownie batter for another 15 seconds until well combined.

5. Pour the batter into a prepared parchment lined 8 X 8 inch baking pan.

6. Spoon the caramel sauce over the batter, then swirl gently into batter with the tip of a toothpick or knife

7. Select Bake and Preheat functions on the Cosori Air Fryer oven, and press Start/Pause.

8. Place the brownies onto the middle rack of the preheated air fryer oven, then press Start/Pause. The air fryer oven will let you know when it is done preheating.

9. Remove the brownies from the oven when done cooking and allow to cool for 1 hour

10. Remove the brownies from the pan, then take off the parchment, cut and serve.

Frozen Brazo de Mercedes

Cooking Time: 1050 minutes   Servings: 8

INGREDIENTS

√ 1 pint vanilla ice cream, softened to room temperature

√ 1 (8 inch) premade graham cracker crust

√ 6 large eggs, yolks and whites separated

√ 7 ounces condensed milk

√ ½ teaspoon vanilla extract

√ ¼ teaspoon cream of tartar

√ 1/3 cup granulated sugar

DIRECTIONS

1. Spread the ice cream on the bottom of the graham cracker crust in an even layer, cover with plastic wrap, and place in the freezer for 8 hours or overnight.

2. Whisk egg yolks and condensed milk over a double boiler continuously for 15 minutes or until the mixture becomes thick.

3. Whisk the vanilla extract into the egg mixture until fully combined.

4. Pass the custard through a fine sieve to remove any clumps.

5. Remove the ice cream and top with the egg yolk mixture, cover with plastic wrap, and place back into the freezer for 2 hours.

6. Beat the egg whites and cream of tartar in a stand mixer on high speed.

7. Add the sugar in slowly once the egg whites begin to foam.

8. Beat the egg whites for two minutes or until they form stiff peaks.

9. Remove the plastic wrap from the pie and top with the beaten egg whites.

10. Select the Preheat function on the Cosori Smart Air Fryer Toaster Oven, adjust temperature to 350°F, and press Start/Pause.

11. Place the pie on the wire rack, then insert the rack at mid position in the preheated air fryer.

12. Select the Bake and Shake functions, adjust time to 15 minutes, and press Start/Pause.

13. Rotate the pie halfway through cooking for even browning. The Shake Reminder will let you know when.

14. Remove when done and place in the fridge for 1 hour, uncovered.

15. Cover the pie, then place in the freezer for 6 hours or overnight.

16. Remove the pie and allow it to rest at room temperature for 10 minutes, then slice and serve.

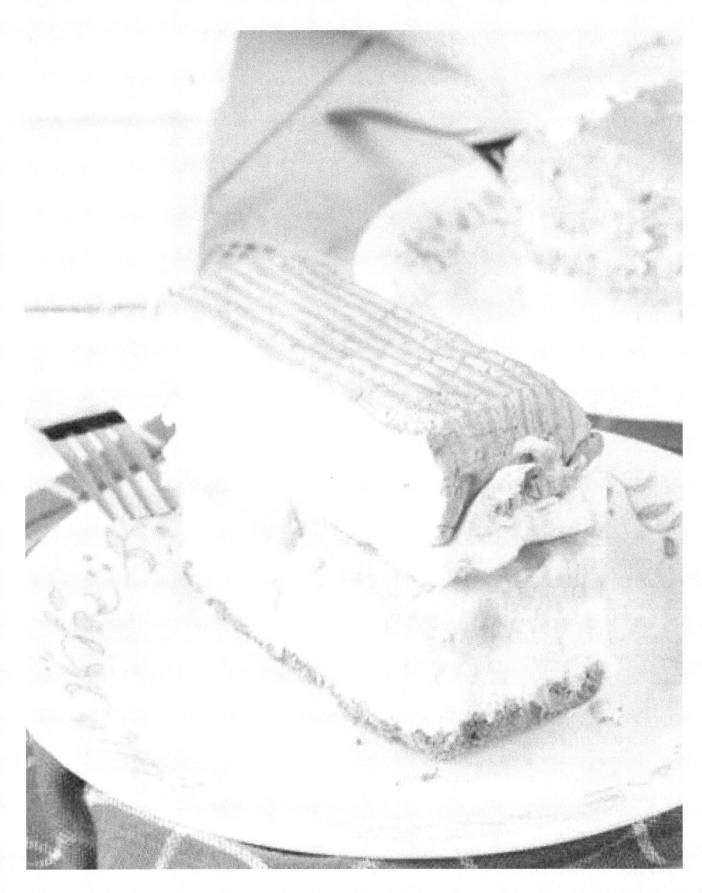

Sesame Seed Balls (Jin Deui)

Cooking Time: 40 minutes   Servings: 4-5

INGREDIENTS

√ 9 ounces red bean paste
√ 2 cups glutinous rice flour
√ 2 tablespoons wheat starch
√ ½ cup granulated sugar
√ A pinch kosher salt
√ 1 teaspoon toasted sesame oil
√ 1½ tablespoons canola oil, plus more for hands
√ ¾ cup warm water
√ ½ cup white sesame seeds

DIRECTIONS

1. Divide the red bean paste into nine 1-ounce balls. Place in the fridge for 5 minutes.
2. Whisk together rice flour, wheat starch, sugar, and kosher salt in a large bowl until well combined.
3. Whisk in the sesame oil and 1½ tablespoons of canola oil into the flour mixture.
4. Stir in the warm water until a dough forms.
5. Knead the dough until smooth, about 2 minutes.
6. Divide the dough into 9 equal balls and lightly coat with canola oil.
7. Flatten the dough balls into 3-inch circles and place a red bean paste ball in the center.
8. Pinch the edges of the dough together to cover the red bean ball and roll to make a ball.
9. Roll each ball into white sesame seeds.
10. Select the Preheat function on the Cosori Air Fryer, adjust to 350°F, and press Start/Pause.
11. Place the sesame seed balls into the preheated air fryer basket lined with parchment paper.
12. Adjust the temperature to 350°F, set time to 25 minutes, and press Start/Pause.
13. Remove from the air fryer and allow it to cool before serving or enjoy hot.

Leche Flan

Cooking Time: 50 minutes   Servings: 4

INGREDIENTS

√ 2/3 cup granulated sugar
√ 4 egg yolks
√ 2/3 cup evaporated milk
√ 2/3 cup sweetened condensed milk
√ ¼ teaspoon vanilla extract
√ A pinch of kosher salt
√ Boiling water

DIRECTIONS

1. Heat the sugar in a saucepan over medium heat until it turns an amber, about 3-5 minutes.
2. Pour the caramel into the oval aluminum pan and set aside.
3. Whisk together egg yolks until well combined. Then whisk in the evaporated milk, sweetened condensed milk, and vanilla extract.
4. Pass the custard through a strainer into a measuring cup and mix in the salt. Set aside.
5. Place the flan into the Cosori cake pan accessory.
6. Select the Preheat function on the Cosori Air Fryer, adjust to 370°F, and press Start/Pause.
7. Place the cake pan into the preheated air fryer basket and fill the cake pan with boiling water just enough to cover the sides of the flan.
8. Adjust the temperature to 370°F, set time for 35 minutes, and press Start/Pause.
9. Place the flan in the fridge for at least 8 hours.
10. Cut along the edges of the flan with a knife to make sure it does not stick when flipping.
11. Flip the leche flan onto a plate and serve.